1 MONTH OF
FREE
READING

at

www.ForgottenBooks.com

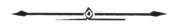

By purchasing this book you are eligible for one month membership to ForgottenBooks.com, giving you unlimited access to our entire collection of over 1,000,000 titles via our web site and mobile apps.

To claim your free month visit:
www.forgottenbooks.com/free59882

ISBN 978-1-5280-6479-8
PIBN 10059882

This book is a reproduction of an important historical work. Forgotten Books uses
state-of-the-art technology to digitally reconstruct the work, preserving the original format
whilst repairing imperfections present in the aged copy. In rare cases, an imperfection in
the original, such as a blemish or missing page, may be replicated in our edition. We do,
however, repair the vast majority of imperfections successfully; any imperfections that
remain are intentionally left to preserve the state of such historical works.

TRANSACTIONS OF THE

SECTION ON

Obstetrics, Gynecology *and* Abdominal Surgery

of the
American Medical Association
at the Sixty-Sixth Annual
Session, held at San Francisco,
June 22 to 25, 1915

AMERICAN MEDICAL ASSOCIATION PRESS
CHICAGO: NINETEEN HUNDRED AND FIFTEEN

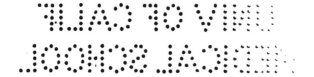

OFFICERS FOR 1914-1915

CHAIRMAN
Thomas S. Cullen - - - - - - - - - Baltimore

VICE CHAIRMAN
George B. Somers - - - - - - - - San Francisco

SECRETARY
Brooke M. Anspach - - - - - - - Philadelphia

EXECUTIVE COMMITTEE
C. Jeff Miller, New Orleans
F. F. Simpson, Pittsburgh
E. Gustav Zinke, Cincinnati

OFFICERS FOR 1915-1916

CHAIRMAN
Edward S. Reynolds - - - - - - - - - Boston

VICE CHAIRMAN
Alfred B. Spalding - - - - - - - - San Francisco

SECRETARY
Brooke M. Anspach - - - - - - - Philadelphia

EXECUTIVE COMMITTEE
F. F. Simpson, Pittsburgh
E. Gustav Zinke, Cincinnati
Thomas S. Cullen, Baltimore

LIST OF OFFICERS

The officers named below have served this Section. That division of practice included under the title of "Obstetrics and Gynecology" was formerly included with branches which now comprise separate sections. The names have been taken from the published records, which are deficient in some cases. It will be appreciated if any additional data are brought to the attention of the Secretary of the American Medical Association.

SECTION ON PRACTICAL MEDICINE AND OBSTETRICS

1860 Chairman, Amos Nourse, Bath, Me.
Secretary, A. K. Gardner, New York.
(Sessions Discontinued on Account of Civil War).

1864 Chairman, B. Fordyce Barker, New York.
Secretary, H. R. Storer, Boston.

1865 Chairman, Z. Pitcher, Detroit.
Secretary, Ellsworth Elliott, New York.

1866 Chairman, L. I. Tefft, Onondaga, N. Y.
Secretary, W. B. Bibbins, New York.

1867 Chairman, M. K. Taylor, Keokuk, Iowa.
Secretary, E. Hall, Auburn, N. Y.

1868 Chairman, R. R. McIlvaine, Cincinnati.
Secretary, C. M. Finch, Portsmouth, Ohio.

1869 Chairman, H. F. Askew, Wilmington, Del.
Secretary, J. C. Hupp, Wheeling, W. Va.

1870 Chairman, Joseph Kammerer, New York.
Secretary, J. C. Jackson, Hartford, Conn.

1871 Chairman, H. R. Storer, Boston.
Secretary, J. K. Bartlett, Milwaukee

1872 Chairman, D. A. O'Donnell, Baltimore.
Secretary, B. F. Dawson, New York.

SECTION ON OBSTETRICS AND DISEASES OF WOMEN AND CHILDREN

1873, Chairman, Theophilus Parvin, Indianapolis.
Secretary, M. A. Pallen, St. Louis.

1874 Chairman, W. H. Byford, Chicago.
Secretary, S. C. Busey, Washington, D. C.

1875 Chairman, S. C. Busey, Washington, D. C.
Secretary, R. Battey, Rome, Ga.

1876 Chairman, J. P. White, New York.
Secretary, R. Battey, Rome, Ga.

1877 Chairman, E. W. Jenks, Detroit.
Secretary, H. O. Marcy, Boston.

1878 Chairman, E. S. Lewis, New Orleans.
Secretary, J. R. Chadwick, Boston.

1879 Chairman, A. H. Smith, Bradford, Pa.
Secretary, R. Battey, Rome, Ga.

SECTION ON OBSTETRICS AND DISEASES OF WOMEN

1880 Chairman, J. R. Chadwick, Boston.
Secretary, J. T. Johnson, Washington, D. C.

1881 Chairman, H. O. Marcy, Boston.
Secretary, C. V. Mottram, Lawrence, Kan.

1882 Chairman, J. K. Bartlett, Milwaukee.
Secretary, G. A. Moses, St. Louis.

1883 Chairman, T. A. Reamy, Cincinnati.
Secretary, J. T. Jelks, Hot Springs, Ark.

1884 Chairman, R. S. Sutton, Pittsburgh.
   Secretary, J. T. Jelks, Hot Springs, Ark.
1885 Chairman, S. C. Gordon, Portland, Maine.
   Secretary, — —, Paine, Texas.
1886 Chairman, F. M. Johnson, Kansas City, Mo.
   Secretary, W. W. Jaggard, Chicago.
1887 Chairman, E. Van De Warker, New York.
   Secretary, E. W. Cushing, Boston.
1888 Chairman, W. H. Wathen, Louisville, Ky.
   Secretary, A. B. Carpenter, Cleveland.
1889 Chairman, W. W. Potter, Buffalo.
   Secretary, J. Hoffman, Philadelphia.
1890 Chairman, C. A. L. Reed, Cincinnati.
   Secretary, H. A. Kelly, Baltimore.
1891 Chairman, E. E. Montgomery, Philadelphia.
   Secretary, F. H. Martin, Chicago.
1892 Chairman, J. M. Duff, Pittsburgh.
   Secretary,
1893 Chairman, J. Eastman, Indianapolis.
   Secretary, G. I. McKelway, Philadelphia.
1894 Chairman, F. H. Martin, Chicago.
   Secretary, X. O. Werder, Pittsburgh.
1895 Chairman, J. T. Johnson, Washington, D. C.
   Secretary, R. Peterson, Grand Rapids, Mich.
1896 Chairman, Milo B. Ward, Topeka, Kan.
   Secretary, G. H. Noble, Atlanta, Ga.
1897 Chairman, Joseph Price, Philadelphia.
   Secretary, C. Lester Hall, Kansas City, Mo.
1898 Chairman, A. H. Cordier, Kansas City, Mo.
   Secretary, W. A. Haggard, Nashville, Tenn.
1899 Chairman, W. E. B. Davis, Birmingham, Ala.
   Secretary, F. F. Lawrence, Columbus, Ohio.
1900 Chairman, H. R. Newman, Chicago.
   Secretary, C. L. Bonifield, Cincinnati.
1901 Chairman, J. H. Carstens, Detroit.
   Secretary, C. L. Bonifield, Cincinnati.

OBSTETRICS AND GYNECOLOGY

1902 Chairman, A. Palmer Dudley, New York.
   Secretary, C. L. Bonifield, Cincinnati.
   Delegates, William H. Humiston, Cleveland; Lewis S. Mc-
   Murtry, Louisville, Ky.
1903 Chairman, L. H. Dunning, Indianapolis.
   Secretary, C. L. Bonifield, Cincinnati.
   Delegates, Edwin S. Ricketts, Cincinnati; E. E. Montgomery,
   Philadelphia.
1904 Chairman, C. L. Bonifield, Cincinnati.
   Secretary, W. P. Manton, Detroit.
   Delegate, W. P. Manton, Detroit.
1905 Chairman, C. S. Bacon, Chicago.
   Secretary, W. P. Manton, Detroit.
   Delegate, Hugo A. Pantzer, Indianapolis.
1906 Chairman, J. W. Bovée, Washington, D. C.
   Secretary, W. P. Manton, Detroit.
   Delegate, Daniel H. Craig, Boston.
1907 Chairman, Walter B. Dorsett, St. Louis.
   Secretary, W. P. Manton, Detroit.
   Delegate, Walter B. Dorsett, St. Louis.
1908 Chairman, W. P. Manton, Detroit.
   Secretary, C. Jeff Miller, New Orleans.
   Delegate, J. T. Watkins.
1909 Chairman, John G. Clark, Philadelphia.
   Vice Chairman, C. C. Frederick, Buffalo.
   Secretary, C. Jeff Miller, New Orleans.
   Delegate, J. H. Carstens, Detroit.

1910 Chairman, Horace G. Wetherill, Denver.
Vice Chairman, Fred J. Taussig, St. Louis.
Secretary, C. Jeff Miller, New Orleans.
Delegate, A. E. Benjamin, Minneapolis.

1911 Chairman, C. Jeff Miller, New Orleans.
Vice Chairman, George B. Somers, San Francisco.
Secretary, F. F. Simpson, Pittsburgh.
Delegate, Horace G. Wetherill, Denver.

OBSTETRICS, GYNECOLOGY AND ABDOMINAL SURGERY

1912 Chairman, F. F. Simpson, Pittsburgh.
Vice Chairman, Joseph B. DeLee, Chicago.
Secretary, Brooke M. Anspach, Philadelphia.
Delegate, Thomas S. Cullen, Baltimore.

1913 Chairman, E. Gustav Zinke, Cincinnati.
Vice Chairman, A. E. Benjamin, Minneapolis.
Secretary, Brooke M. Anspach, Philadelphia.
Delegate, R. R. Smith, Grand Rapids, Mich.

1914 Chairman, Thomas S. Cullen, Baltimore.
Vice Chairman, George B. Somers, San Francisco.
Secretary, Brooke M. Anspach, Philadelphia.
Delegate, Channing W. Barrett, Chicago.

1915 Chairman, Edward S. Reynolds, Boston.
Vice Chairman, Alfred B. Spalding, San Francisco.
Secretary, Brooke M. Anspach, Philadelphia.
Delegate, P. Brookes Bland, Philadelphia.

CONTENTS

PROCEEDINGS OF THE SECTION

The section was called to order at 2 p. m. by Dr. Alfred B. Spalding, San Francisco.

On account of the illness of the chairman, Dr. Thomas S. Cullen, Baltimore, and vice chairman, Dr. George B. Somers, San Francisco, the section unanimously elected Dr. S. H. Buteau, Oakland, Calif., to act as chairman, and Dr. Spalding was elected secretary.

The address of the chairman, Dr. Thomas S. Cullen, Baltimore, entitled "The Relation of Surgery, Gynecology and Obstetrics to the Public," was read by Dr. Horace G. Wetherill, Denver. No discussion.

Dr. J. Morris Slemons, San Francisco, read a paper on "Placental Bacteremia." Discussed by Drs. E. E. Montgomery of Philadelphia, and Henry O. Marcy, Boston.

Dr. E. E. Montgomery, Philadelphia, read a paper on "Abortion." Discussed by Drs. Alfred B. Spalding, San Francisco; John Osborn Polak, Brooklyn; C. Lester Hall, Kansas City, Mo.; S. M. Clark, New Orleans; Horace G. Wetherill, Denver, and E. E. Montgomery, Philadelphia.

Dr. Henry O. Marcy, Boston, read a paper on "The Histogenesis of the Reproductive Processes in Mammals." Discussed by Dr. E. E. Montgomery, Philadelphia.

The following papers were read as a symposium on anesthesia in labor:

Dr. Carl H. Davis, Chicago: "Advantages of Nitrous Oxid Analgesia in Obstetrics over the Freiburg Method."

Dr. John Osborn Polak, Brooklyn: "The Appreciation and Limitations of Morphin-Scopolamin Amnesia in Obstetrics."

These two papers were discussed by Drs. Walter E. Libby, San Francisco; W. Francis B. Wakefield, San Francisco; J. C. Litzenberg, Minneapolis; C. G. Parsons, Denver; Carl L. Hoag, San Francisco; L. I. Breitstein, San Francisco; M. W. Kapp, San José, Calif.; E. M. Lazard, Los Angeles; L. M. Gates, Scranton, Pa.; Hugh S. Mount, Oregon City, Ore.; W. R. Livingston, Oxnard, Calif.; Carl H. Davis, Chicago, and J. O. Polak, Brooklyn.

The following officers were elected: chairman, Dr. Edward J. Reynolds, Boston; vice chairman, Dr. Alfred B. Spalding, San Francisco; secretary, Dr. Brooke M. Anspach, Philadelphia; member of the House of Delegates, Dr. P. Brooke Bland, Philadelphia.

Dr. Howard Canning Taylor, New York, read a paper on "Tuberculosis of the Uterine Appendages." Discussed by Drs. Philemon E. Truesdale, Fall River, Mass.; J. E. Engstad, Minneapolis; O. W. Hall, Kansas City, Mo.; E. E. Montgomery, Philadelphia; S. M. D. Clark, New Orleans, and Howard Canning Taylor, New York.

Dr. W. D. Haggard, Nashville, Tenn., read a paper on "Application of Various Theories in the Practical Management of Peritonitis." Discussed by Drs. W. B. Brinsmade, Brooklyn; J. O. Polak, Brooklyn; Edward Reynolds, Boston; Joseph B. DeLee, Chicago, and H. O. Pantzer, Indianapolis.

Dr. L. G. Bowers, Dayton, O., read a paper on "Pelvic Infection and the Application of Drainage." Discussed by Drs. S. M. D. Clark, New Orleans; H. W. Gibbons, San Francisco, and L. G. Bowers, Dayton, O.

Dr. Alfred B. Spalding, San Francisco, read a paper on "Relative Frequency of Ectopic Gestation." Discussed by Dr. Joseph B. DeLee, Chicago, and Alfred B. Spalding, San Francisco.

Dr. Edward Reynolds, Boston, read a paper on "The Prognosis of Sterility." Discussed by Drs. J. O. Polak, Brooklyn; Joseph B. DeLee, Chicago; H. O. Pantzer, Indianapolis, and Edward Reynolds, Boston.

The following papers were read as a symposium on the treatment of cancer of the uterus and rectum by radium:

Dr. Henry Schmitz, Chicago: "Primary Results of Radium Therapy on Uterine and Rectal Cancers."

Drs. Curtis F. Burnam and Howard A. Kelly, Baltimore: "Radium in the Treatment of Carcinomas of the Cervix Uteri and Vagina."

These two papers were discussed by Drs. J. F. Percy, Galesburg, Ill.; S. M. D. Clark, New Orleans; Henry Schmitz, Chicago, and Curtis F. Burnam, Baltimore.

THURSDAY, JUNE 24—AFTERNOON

Dr. Horace G. Wetherill, Denver, read a paper on "Subinfection from Foci in the Pelvis and Abdomen." Discussed by Drs. Carl H. Davis, Chicago, and Alfred B. Spalding, San Francisco.

Dr. W. Wayne Babcock, Philadelphia, read a paper on "Cholecystectomy and Cholecystic Toxemia." Discussed by Dr. Robert C. Coffey, Portland, Ore., and W. Wayne Babcock, Philadelphia.

Dr. P. E. Truesdale, Fall River, Mass., read a paper on "The Pylorus: Observations Noted in Association with

Gastro-Intestinal Lesions." Discussed by Drs. Frederick Murphy, St. Louis, and Max Einhorn, New York.

Dr. Robert C. Coffey, Portland, Ore., read a paper on "The Significance of the Fixation of Certain Abdominal Organs in the Human Body." Discussed by Drs. Max Einhorn, New York; Albert Goldspohn, Chicago; A. N. Creadick, Portland, Ore.; H. O. Pantzer, Indianapolis, and R. C. Coffey, Portland, Ore.

Alexius McGlannan, Baltimore, read a paper on "Intestinal Obstruction." Discussed by Drs. Draper, New York, and Alex. McGlannan, New York.

On motion of Dr. Wetherill, duly seconded, the secretary was requested to express to Dr. George B. Somers, San Francisco, the regret of the section at his inability to attend the meeting.

On motion of Dr. Wetherill, duly seconded, the section expressed its appreciation, by rising vote,.to Dr. Buteau for acting as chairman, and Dr. Spalding, as secretary, and for the very able manner in which they had performed these duties.

THE RELATION OF OBSTETRICS, GYNE-COLOGY AND ABDOMINAL SURGERY TO THE PUBLIC WELFARE *

THOMAS S. CULLEN, M.D.
BALTIMORE

To be selected chairman of any section of the American Medical Association is an honor which a man may be proud of; to be named the presiding officer of this very important section was a compliment I little dreamed of, and I am deeply grateful for the confidence placed in me.

An artist from time to time steps back from his easel to get a good view of the painting he has in progress. The business man at regular periods takes stock to see what are his assets and liabilities. We in like manner should at frequent intervals leave our labors and, figuratively speaking, ascend the mountain peak whence we may overlook the plain of our daily labors and may be able not only to see what has been accomplished but also to detect the weak spots, the points at which our endeavors have fallen short.

In the time allotted to the presiding officer I shall briefly give a panoramic view of obstetrics, gynecology and abdominal surgery as I saw them twenty-five years ago, and shall then compare them with the same branches of medicine as we find them today.

THE OBSTETRICS, GYNECOLOGY AND ABDOMINAL SURGERY OF TWENTY-FIVE YEARS AGO

Obstetrics.—In many localities, obstetrics and diseases of children were still linked together, the accoucheur not only looking after the child at birth but

---

* Chairman's Address.

also attending to it during its early years. With the gradual awakening to the fact that childrens' sore throats were often streptococcic in origin, that a case of puerperal fever might follow the too close association of the obstetrician with a case of scarlet fever, that diphtheria was due to a definite germ; and further, with the rapid development of pediatrics into an important specialty, it was deemed wiser to separate the practice of diseases of children from that of obstetrics. Thus at the time of my graduation, just a quarter of a century ago, we had one relatively small, although splendidly equipped, lying-in hospital in a city of about 125,000. It was presided over by a most capable physician who limited his work almost exclusively to obstetrics. He not only obtained excellent results but was also a most able teacher—a man who left his impress on all those who had the privilege of his instruction. Few obstetric teachers did more conscientious work than did Adam Wright who, I am glad to say, is still with us.

Gynecology.—In my student days the pupils learned that there were anteversions, anteflexions, retroversions and retroflexions and that some of the displacements might be relieved by appropriate pessaries. We were told of erosions of the cervix and had the value of zinc chlorid or Churchill's tincture of iodin as the proper agents in the treatment for such conditions drilled into us day after day. Much stress was laid on laceration of the cervix, and many repairs were done. Now and again a torn perineum was also treated surgically.

Abdominal gynecologic operations were limited almost entirely to the removal of large ovarian cysts. An occasional myomatous uterus was removed, but the fatality in this class of cases was so high that the operation was rarely attempted. We occasionally heard of cancer of the cervix or of carcinoma of the body of the uterus, but the only operative procedures we were familiar with for this dread disease were curettage, and cauterization of the carcinomatous cervix. To entirely remove the uterus for this condition was not thought of.

Abdominal Surgery.—Fractures were well handled and the surgery of the outside of the body and lateral lithotomy were successfully and dextrously performed, but abdominal operations were undertaken with great trepidation. Surgery of the stomach was rarely if ever seen. Gallstones were not removed, and I have seen a leading medical consultant watch an appendix abscess for over a week, hoping that it would soon rupture externally. The appendix was rarely, if ever, removed. As an intern in the medical ward, I watched a patient with a perforation due to typhoid ulcer for seven days — until the woman's death — when the diagnosis was verified at necropsy. One of the abdominal cases most vividly impressed on my mind was that of a thin, elderly man with definite intestinal obstruction. He was in good condition when he entered the hospital, but gradually grew worse and died after a few days. Through a small hole in the mesentery a short loop of the small bowel had passed. Even at necropsy this loop could be pulled back with the utmost ease.

The experiences I have just related occurred in a large institution presided over by most capable medical men and surgeons. I have mentioned them in no spirit of criticism whatsoever. Their modes of treatment were similar to those carried out in nearly all the hospitals throughout the land, and the same hospital today is doing first-class up-to-date surgery. To you who have been in practice these many years our former failures are too well known. For those of you who have graduated within the last fifteen or twenty years it is well to realize what great strides have been made in abdominal surgery and gynecology during the last two decades.

I' will now pass to the consideration of the obstetrics, gynecology and abdominal surgery of today — a theme with which you are much more familiar.

Obstetrics.—The recognition of the absolute necessity of a thorough obstetric training is realized throughout the land, and adequate lying-in hospitals are being furnished in numerous cities — not in all, I am sorry to say. The medical students in many of the schools not only see a large number of births but individually must look after a certain number of obstetric patients. In addition, they receive a systematic course of instruction in obstetric pathology. The fundamental handling of obstetric cases has naturally not undergone so marked a change as has the treatment of gynecologic and abdominal cases, because gynecology and abdominal surgery are relatively new fields.

Gynecology.—To the older members of the profession the "gynecologist" may still suggest the pessary and Churchill's tincture of iodin; and it is hard for them to realize that at the present day the surgical procedures dealing with the perineum and of the pelvis are on just as firm and stable a basis as is the surgery of other portions of the body. The fundamental knowledge we owe in large measure to the pathologist, who has traced out the pathologic conditions from the beginning and has indicated the paths along which the disease may travel. For example, given a patient with a gonorrheal infection, we have only to remember that the germ comes from without. It may invade Skene's glands and the urethra; it may implicate Bartholin's glands, and then in succession the vagina, the cervix, the body of the uterus, the tubes and finally the pelvic peritoneum. Knowing the mode of progression of this infection, we can the more intelligently adopt the appropriate medical or surgical procedure.

We now know that a perineal operation alone may be of little value in the treatment of a case of prolapsus, and that failure will often follow if we do not at the same time shorten the round or uterosacral ligaments.

Our knowledge of tubal and ovarian diseases is sufficiently accurate to enable us in many cases to do conservative operations instead of unsexing the woman. Our studies of uterine tumors supplemented by an improved technic now enables us to do a supravaginal hysterectomy with little risk to the patient. When a patient complains of uterine hemorrhage we can usually within twenty-four to forty-eight hours tell her with a surprising degree of accuracy the cause of this hemorrhage.

Twenty-five years ago cancer of the uterus was nearly always fatal; today it is far more amenable to treatment. Fully two-thirds of all cancers of the body of the uterus can be permanently cured if operated on early, and some surgeons have been able to report 25 per cent. of their patients operated on for cancer of the cervix as well five years later. When the splendid work being done by the American Society for the Control of Cancer, the Cancer Campaign Committee of the Clinical Congress of Surgeons, and the Cancer Committee of the Council on Health and Public Instruction of the American Medical Association has sunk deep into the minds of the laity of this country, the results will be even more encouraging.

I might dwell at length on the fundamental advances made by Howard A. Kelly and others in the methods of studying diseases of the bladder and kidney, but with these far-reaching contributions to gynecology you are also thoroughly familiar.

Abdominal Surgery.—The advances in abdominal surgery during the last twenty-five years have been so marked that they are almost overwhelming. Even fifteen years ago the ruptured appendix with or without a peritonitis was exceedingly common. The general practitioner has become such a champion of early operation that in many clinics, if the appendix happens to be ruptured when the abdomen is opened, he at once chides himself for any possible delay that may have occurred. Just here I should like to say that I am thoroughly convinced that in the past the one or more doses of calomel and the subsequent dose of salts have been in a large measure responsible for the appalling conditions found at operation. Thus far I have never seen a patient die who was operated on for appendicitis before the appendix ruptured.

Twenty-five years ago few operations were performed on the gallbladder. Now if there be any prolonged discomfort or distress in this region, the gallbladder is promptly explored, in the vast majority of cases with permanent relief. The stomach washings, which were so prevalent even a decade ago, have in a large measure disappeared as a result of the prompt removal of the appendix or drainage of the gallbladder according to the nature of the case, and are, as a rule, resorted to only when it is necessary to make gastric analyses.

Operations on the stomach were formerly rarely undertaken. Now gastro-enterostomy is a common and relatively safe procedure. Ulcers are removed, strictures relieved, and where carcinoma is suspected, an exploratory operation is done at the earliest possible moment.

Inseparably coupled with the advances made in this branch of surgery are the names of William J. Mayo, John M. T. Finney, W. L. Rodman and many others.

Intestinal surgery twenty-five years ago was in the experimental stage, and we in this country are indebted to Nicholas Senn, William S. Halsted, Franklin P. Mall, John B. Murphy and others for their pioneer experimental work in this direction. When intestinal obstruction develops, we do not now fold our hands, saying that the case is hopeless, but at once do an enterostomy and, when the patient has improved sufficiently, hunt for the cause of the obstruction if nature has not in the meantime corrected it. I might describe the advances made in the surgery of other parts of the abdomen, but with these you are also familiar. The great strides made in abdominal surgery and in gynecology have of course been rendered possible by the fundamental labors of Louis Pasteur and Joseph Lister, and by those of Robert Koch,[1] who in 1878 published his important paper on the causation of diseases from wound infection. Dr. W. W. Ford,[2] in speaking of this work says:

In this paper Koch puts forward clearly the exact state of knowledge on the subject of surgical infections; he explains the difficulties which had to be overcome in working out their etiology and describes the results which others before him had achieved.

To those of you who have had a share in this great advance it must have been the source of the utmost satisfaction. To have lived during this period has been a great privilege. The progress in abdominal surgery of the last twenty-five years has without a doubt been greater than will ever occur in a similar period. The immediate death rate has been reduced from about 25 per cent. to 2 or 3 per cent.; thus, if we temporarily relieved all patients we could reduce our mortality only 3 per cent. more.

There is no reason, however, why we should be in the least complacent. Many of our patients suffering from tuberculous peritonitis are only temporarily relieved. We are helpless in our cases of general peritoneal carcinosis, and many cases of cancer of the stomach, intestine, uterus and ovaries are beyond our control. There is still much to be accomplished.

---

1. Koch, Robert: Untersuchungen über die Aetiologie der Wundinfektionskrankheiten, 1878.
2. Ford, W. W.: Johns Hopkins Hosp. Bull., 1911, xxii, 420.

THE ALIGNMENT OF OBSTETRICS, GYNECOLOGY AND ABDOMINAL SURGERY

With the rapid development in these three branches, new problems have arisen, and it may be well for us to consider briefly the relation that these three branches in question should bear to one another.

Obstetrics.—A thorough knowledge of this art is infinitely more important to the student than is a clear understanding of gynecology. The vast majority of medical students after graduation attend obstetric cases. These young general practitioners, if living in a fair-sized town or city, may when in trouble be able to consult with an obstetric expert, but often the practitioner's time for temporizing is so limited that he must rely absolutely on his own initiative. The physician living in the small town or in the country must pilot his patient through the dangerous shoals, relying entirely on the knowledge he has obtained from his former teachers, coupled with his own liberal supply of good horse-sense.

Gynecologic cases rarely call for such speedy treatment. If the general practitioner is uncertain as to his diagnosis and does not know just what to do, he can, as a rule, temporize for a day or two and in the meantime have a consultation with a gynecologist. Furthermore, most of the gynecologic patients are well enough to journey to the city to see the consultant at his office or at the hospital.

In obstetric cases the vast majority of the physicians are obliged to take full charge of the case irrespective of its gravity; hence the absolute necessity of our turning out graduates of medicine thoroughly grounded in the theory and practice of obstetrics. Dr. J. Whitridge Williams[3] has given us a most comprehensive summary of the obstetric teaching in this country, and

3. Williams, J. Whitridge: Has the American Gynecological Society Done Its Part in the Advancement of Obstetrical Knowledge, THE JOURNAL A. M. A., June 6, 1914, p. 1767.

pointed out in no uncertain terms the growing need for better methods and facilities.

In years past some of the prominent members of the profession tried to confine their labors to obstetrics and gynecology. A few succeeded, but as their practices increased the majority either became obstetricians or confined their work almost entirely to gynecology. This was but natural, as these two branches cannot be well handled together. In fact, obstetrics is similar to emergency surgery. No one can decide exactly when the birth will take place, nor can he determine with any degree of accuracy how long the labor will last.

Supposing the surgeon who practices these two specialties arranges for four abdominal operations for tomorrow morning, and that just as he is leaving for the hospital to operate he receives an urgent call to come and see one of his primiparas who is in labor. If this confinement lasts several hours, these four operations have to be postponed, the postponement causing much added anxiety not only to the four patients but also to the various relatives. A few such delays as this, and the friends of the patients will naturally look for surgeons that can be relied on to fulfil their engagements promptly. In a way this is very unfair to the obstetrician, inasmuch as the delay has been in no way his fault; and yet the fact remains that it has been due entirely to an attempt on his part to combine two specialties that are not compatible with one another.

Again, let our surgeon arrange for a Wertheim operation on a cancer patient for tomorrow morning. This is without doubt one of the hardest abdominal procedures. The surgeon should be in the pink of condition, and it should be his first operation for the day. During the night he is called out to an obstetric case and is detained several hours. If he operates in the cancer case on schedule time, is he doing justice to himself or to his patient?

Is there any wonder that many physicians have given up this combination of obstetric and gynecologic practice? When asking your young medical men what line of work they are doing, they will often say that they are at the present time paying particular attention to obstetrics, hoping later to enter the surgical ranks; and many of the older men, who have good obstetric practices, are relegating that work to associates as their surgical practice increases. Do you blame them? Few there are who would not do likewise. When we look at the subject squarely, it is clearly evident that the obstetric specialist is the true missionary of the medical profession, and the most unselfish member in its ranks. Even though he be the head of his department, his time is not his own and there is no hour of the day or night when he may not be called.

From what Dr. Williams has told us, the obstetric training in America is not what it should be. Is it going to be improved if the head of the department, whenever possible, naturally but gradually drifts over into surgery, leaving the obstetric teaching, both practical and theoretical, largely in the hands of his associates? It is the duty of this Association to so improve the facilities and opportunities of the obstetrician that he will devote all his energies to the furtherance of this all-important branch of medicine. I say "all-important," because on his teaching and practice depends in large measure the life and happiness of the coming citizens of this land.

With the rapid progress in medicine and surgery, the needs of the obstetric clinics have been in large measure relegated to the background. All large hospitals should have capacious and well equipped lying-in departments and I feel confident that in the near future even the smaller towns will erect up-to-date lying-in hospitals.

The young obstetrician in his preparatory training should include a thorough knowledge of medicine, pathology and bacteriology, and should also serve as a surgical assistant for a relatively long period before taking up his work in obstetrics. When he starts out as a trained obstetrician, he should be able at once to meet any abdominal or perineal surgical emergency that he may encounter. The obstetrician has the right to demand that every possible facility be afforded him. Not until this fact is so thoroughly realized that it is acted on by the profession, will the best men be content to remain in this important but most arduous field of labor.

If it could be so arranged that all private obstetric patients were delivered in maternity hospitals, the wear and tear on the obstetrician would be greatly lessened, and he would then have more time to work out the many important and still unsolved problems connected with this branch of medicine. Some of the problems extend over into other branches. Menstruation is undoubtedly one of these. Much has been said about it, but thus far little is known. It seems to me that it will require the combined labors of the anatomist, physiologist, physiologic chemist, obstetrician and gynecologist, together with much experimental work, before our knowledge on this subject becomes in any way complete.

Gynecology and Abdominal Surgery.—In the early days in this country travel was confined to the seaboard and rivers. If one wished to go from Baltimore to New York, the journey was made almost exclusively by water, and was one extending over several days. Gradually paths were carried back into the wilderness for a short distance, and later primitive roads were built and finally good stage roads. It was then possible to travel by fast relaying from Baltimore to New York in a few days. Now our express trains require four hours between these two points.

The progress in abdominal surgery and gynecology bears a striking resemblance to the gradual evolution in travel. In the beginning, only the outer surface of the abdomen and the vagina could be operated on. At a later date an occasional excursion was made into the abdomen, as successfully carried out by McDowell. With the epoch-making discovery of asepsis, the motive power was furnished, enabling us to traverse all parts of the abdomen. Since that date the "civilizing" influences have been gradually extended until the abdomen and its contents are fairly well understood: There still remain, however, a certain number of dismal swamps and everglades.

The greater part of gynecology deals with the surgery of the lower abdomen. Sometimes the operation is entirely confined to an exploration of the abdomen, but frequently, as in prolapsus cases, in order that a satisfactory result may be obtained, it is also necessary to carry out some vaginal operation in connection with that in the pelvis. Where large tumors exist, the confines of the pelvis are temporarily carried far up into the abdomen, occasionally as high as the liver, and now and then the intestines are densely adherent and may require resection.

In a no mean percentage of the cases, digestive disturbances are associated with a pelvic lesion, and naturally require investigation at the time of operation. The surgeon, who largely confines his labors to the upper abdomen, not infrequently finds pelvic lesions which he little suspected before the abdomen was opened.

If the gynecologist confines his work entirely to the pelvis, he will not infrequently overlook lesions in the upper abdomen, and the surgeon in like manner will miss serious pelvic trouble.

When you or I take a watch to the jeweler, we expect him to overhaul it thoroughly, examining all portions of its mechanism. If he returns it saying that the mainspring which was broken has been repaired, but the watch still will not go, we are naturally dissatisfied and will try a more competent man. If we do not carefully explore the abdomen in all cases, we are bound to overlook many little-dreamed-of pathologic conditions — conditions that will still render the patient uncomfortable.

Suppose I have done some pelvic operation and have overlooked gallstones or a duodenal ulcer. The patient will usually be far from well and will in a few weeks or months decide to call in a man capable of properly treating the upper abdominal lesion. What does this lack of preparedness on my part entail for the patient? Twice the length of time in the hospital, twice the amount of pain, twice the amount of hospital expense and two operation fees, not to speak of the added risk of the second operation. This is an age of economy, an age of short cuts, and an age when by-products are utilized to the limit. It will not be long before the laity will demand that any one who enters an abdomen must be capable of doing everything necessary in that abdomen, and in those cases in which, on account of the lesion present, a second operation is required, it will be necessary for us to explain carefully just why the abdomen must be opened again. Some one will say, "This is all very well; you should make an accurate diagnosis beforehand." This might be perfectly plausible if the anterior abdominal wall were made of plate glass, but even then, as we all know, sometimes, when the abdomen has been opened, it requires considerable search to find the exact location of the trouble. Now and then, when visiting the clinics of well-known surgeons, I cannot help looking with a twinge of wicked pleasure on seeing that their diagnoses do not always tally with the findings — it makes me feel thoroughly at home. The only abdominal surgeon who makes no mistakes in diagnosis is either the one who has no practice or the one who has given up the scalpel.

In recent years, business men have been greatly aided by economy or efficiency experts. Strangers come in, look over the business and see where, by more efficient methods, more may be accomplished, often with diminished labor. If we called in such an expert, what would he say? In the first place, he would point out that it is not necessary for two classes of surgeons to work in one abdomen — a space the confines of which nature has so well defined. In the second place, he would say to both the surgeon of the upper abdomen and to the surgeon of the lower abdomen: "You have spent long years in preparing yourselves for doing abdominal surgery, you have mastered the fundamentals of medicine, you have a good knowledge of bacteriology and pathology and have perfected yourselves in the methods of operation; and yet, because one pelvis happens to contain a small round muscular body with two smaller bodies on the sides, one of you confines your work in large measure to men, the other to women. You are only running half capacity. There is absolutely no reason whatsoever why you should not both do abdominal surgery in the two sexes. It is practically the same, the only difference being that there is no operation in abdominal surgery that can compare in difficulty with a complicated Wertheim operation for cancer of the cervix." After seventeen years' experience in abdominal surgery in men and women, I myself am absolutely convinced that pelvic surgery offers many more difficulties and is harder of execution than is the surgery of the upper abdomen.

THE TRAINING OF THE ABDOMINAL SURGEON

Every man who aims to make abdominal surgery his life work should have a most thorough training in general medicine. He will then not forget that pain in the right iliac fossa does not always mean appendicitis. He will know that occasionally this soreness is present in an early stage of typhoid fever. He will remember that there is such a thing as lead colic and that in children severe abdominal pain may be the precursor of a pneumonia. A thorough knowledge of this most fundamental and broadest branch of medicine will save him from many pitfalls.

In addition to his course in general pathology he should have an extensive knowledge of the pathology of all the abdominal structures. The abdominal surgeon of the future must be a well-grounded pathologist; two years in the necropsy room would be of inestimable value to him. Then he should pay particular attention to the bacterial flora associated with the various abdominal lesions. He has now finished his apprenticeship, and should become an assistant of an abdominal surgeon. Here he will not only learn the various operative procedures and perfect himself in these, but he will also become experienced in the preparatory and after-treatment of the patients. The after-treatment, by the way, is of great importance, the postoperative journey often being rough and tempestuous, or relatively smooth, according to the manner in which the assistant handles the case. After several years spent in this way, the assistant is thoroughly competent to start out on his career. The surgery of the United States has made wonderful strides during the last decade. We must prepare ourselves to become the graduate school for the world.

CONCLUSION

In the brief time at my disposal I have hastily scanned the salient points relating to obstetrics, gynecology and abdominal surgery, the subjects treated in our section. Necessarily much has been omitted. The points that I want to leave with you are:

1. Obstetrics must be made more attractive, so that those entering this branch will not be tempted to leave it for less laborious fields.

2. Any surgeon opening the abdomen should be capable of doing everything necessary in that abdomen. In other words, gynecology and abdominal surgery logically belong together.

3. This realignment of abdominal surgery is absolutely necessary if we are to accomplish the maximum amount of good for the patient.

20 East Eager Street.

PLACENTAL BACTEREMIA

J. MORRIS SLEMONS, M.D.
Professor of Obstetrics and Gynecology, Yale Medical School
NEW HAVEN, CONN.

When the fetus is stillborn or the infant dies within a few days after its birth, frequently we are unable to determine the cause of death. This fact has been emphasized in the statistical analyses recently published from two American institutions. At the Sloane Hospital for Women[1] among 10,000 consecutive confinements there were 429 stillbirths and 291 infants which died within two weeks after they were born. Reviewing an equal number of confinements at the Johns Hopkins Hospital, J. Whitridge Williams[2] found 705 cases of stillbirth and early infant death. The fetal mortality in these clinics, it would seem, is practically identical. And in both series of statistics it is instructive to find that, although careful clinical observations and postmortem examinations were made, the cause of death was not ascertained in roundly 20 per cent. of the fatal cases.

Some time ago my attention was called to a cause of fetal death not widely appreciated and one which is left out of account in the reports just quoted. Whenever membranes rupture prematurely and the labor is prolonged, especially if repeated vaginal examinations are made, bacterial invasion of the placenta—placental bacteremia—may occur. This complication constitutes a serious danger for the fetus. Its relative importance as a factor in infant mortality is difficult to estimate but its practical significance is certain.

1. Holt, L. Emmett, and Babbitt, Ellen C.: Institutional Mortality of the Newborn, The Journal A. M. A., Jan. 23, 1915, p. 287.
2. Williams, J. Whitridge: Limitations and Possibilities of Prenatal Care, The Journal A. M. A., Jan. 9, 1915, p. 95.

With reference to this question I have studied five hundred consecutive confinements under my care while connected with the University of California Hospital. Including infants over 40 cm. long the mortality was 5.4 per cent. (27 cases). The infant was stillborn in 21 cases; it died on the second day in 3, on the fourth in 2, and on the ninth in 1 case. A necropsy was performed in every instance. The causes of death were as follows:

	Cases	Per Cent.
Syphilis	7	26
Birth injury	6	22
Premature separation of placenta	4	15
Placental bacteremia	3	11
Congenital heart lesion	2	7
Enlarged thymus	1	3
Toxemia pregnancy	1	3
Undetermined	3	11

A number of well-known factors combine to explain why the fetal mortality is higher in case labor is prolonged. With 62 of my patients labor lasted longer than twenty-four hours and in this group 8 fetal deaths occurred (13 per cent.). Three of the deaths were due to placental bacteremia. The mothers of these infants were not seriously ill and at the end of two weeks were discharged from the hospital in good health. Such results, it will be made clear, are not always to be expected. But before considering the experience of other observers I may summarize the histories of my cases, giving only the facts pertinent to the problem under discussion.

CASE 1.—Primipara; aged 20; generally contracted rachitic pelvis with diagonal conjugate measuring 11 cm. Presentation right occipitoposterior. Duration of labor twenty-eight hours: membranes ruptured six hours before delivery by midforceps. Several vaginal examinations were made but the number was not recorded. Temperature during labor, 37.8 C. (100 F.); pulse, 70. Highest puerperal temperature, 37 C. (98.6 F.); pulse, 98.

The child, 48 cm. long, weighed 3,080 gm. It was easily resuscitated. Death occurred on the third day. At necropsy the umbilical stump was dry and clean. The abdomen contained 250 c.c. of seropurulent fluid which showed streptococci in cover slips. There were subpleural ecchymoses over the left lung, but no intracranial hemorrhage and no meningitis. The brain was normal.

Sections of the placenta and umbilical cord stained with hematoxylin and eosin were normal. Sections of the placenta stained by the Gram-Weigert method showed a few streptococci just beneath the amnion in the neighborhood of the fetal blood vessels. Bacteria were not demonstrated in the cord.

CASE 2.—Primipara; aged 23; normal pelvis. Presentation left occipito-anterior. Labor began with rupture of the membranes and after forty-five hours terminated normally. Six vaginal examinations were made. Temperature during labor, 38 C.; pulse, 108. Highest puerperal temperature was 38.2 C.; pulse, 110.

The child, 52 cm. long, weighed 3,540 gm. Resuscitation was difficult. Death occurred at the end of forty-eight hours. Shortly after its birth the infant bled from the mouth, and later patches of purpura appeared over the head, buttocks, scrotum and right knee. At necropsy a small blood clot was found on the parietal peritoneum adjacent to the umbilical vessels and another beneath the liver. The peritoneal cavity contained about 10 c.c. of uncoagulated blood but none was found in the intestines. There was no blood in the pleural cavity. Several hemorrhages the size of a pinhead were found at the base of each lung.

Sections of the placenta stained with hematoxylin and eosin were normal but the umbilical cord was infiltrated with leukocytes, most pronouncedly in the neighborhood of the vein. Stained by the Gram-Weigert method streptococci were demonstrated in the amniotic and chorionic connective tissue near the fetal surface of the placenta. Streptococci were also present in the cord.

CASE 3.—Primipara; aged 38; normal pelvis. Presentation left occipito-anterior. Membranes ruptured when the cervix was dilated 5 cm., twenty-four hours before delivery was effected by midforceps. Temperature during labor, 37.8 C.; pulse, 106. Highest puerperal temperature, 38.5 C. (101.3 F.); pulse, 115.

The child, 50 cm. long, weighed 2,980 gm. For an hour before delivery the fetal heart sounds were not heard. The necropsy findings were negative except for a small cerebral hemorrhage beneath the left occipital lobe.

Sections of the placenta showed partial thrombosis of many of the vessels which pass over the fetal surface of the placenta. Large numbers of bacteria were demonstrated in the amnion covering the placenta and in the underlying chorionic connective tissue. Streptococci and also a short, stout bacillus, resembling the gas bacillus, were present. A few streptococci were found in the intervillous spaces but the chorionic villi were normal. A typical mixed thrombus almost completely blocked the umbilical vein. It contained streptococci as did also the wall of the vein and the surrounding Whartonian jelly. The walls of the umbilical arteries were slightly infiltrated with leukocytes but no bacteria were demonstrated there.

In all these cases organisms were demonstrated in the subamniotic connective tissue where they came in contact with the large fetal blood vessels which cross the surface of the placenta. In one instance it was possible to demonstrate bacteria in the act of penetrating the walls of these vessels. It is also noteworthy that in every case the epithelium which covers the villi was intact, the capillaries within the villi were of normal appearance, and no bacteria were found either on the surface or in the interior of the villi. Evidently the infection did not proceed from the maternal circulation and did not pass through the walls of the villi. The bacteria entered the placenta by way of the amniotic membrane. Most frequently, as in these cases, placental bacteremia depends on the infection of the amniotic fluid; and generally the latter complication occurs because the membranes rupture prematurely, labor is prolonged, and repeated vaginal examinations are made.

From a knowledge of the anatomy of pregnancy it is obvious that, at least theoretically, the infection of the amniotic fluid is possible by three routes; (1) organisms may pass from the maternal circulation across the decidua, the chorion, and the amnion; (2) they may travel from the peritoneal cavity down the fallopian tubes, or (3) they may ascend from the vagina through the cervical canal. In a series of animal experiments the progress of an infection along each of these paths has been demonstrated by Hellendall,[3] but only the third has a broad, practical significance in human pathology. It has not been established that the other routes ever play a rôle

3. Hellendall: Beitr. z. Geburtsh. u. Gynäk., 1906, x, 320.

except under conditions that have been imposed experimentally. And yet, it is possible in human beings that hematogenous infection of the amniotic fluid may be the result of a maternal septicemia; and also that in case of acute inflammation of the appendix during pregnancy the responsible organisms may find their way down one of the fallopian tubes. At all events, in the cases I have observed, neither septicemia, appendicitis, nor peritonitis existed; on the other hand, ideal conditions prevailed for infection of the amniotic fluid by the vaginal route.

When the membranes have ruptured, an increased liability to infection is apparent; and some have taught that bacterial invasion of the amniotic cavity occurred while the membranes were intact. The evidence favoring the latter possibility, however, is not conclusive, as it has never been confirmed by bacteriologic examination. In the cases recorded by Lehmann, Carpentier, Brieglet, Lendanthal[4] and others, the foul smelling decomposed amniotic fluid which escaped when the membranes ruptured may have been due, as these observers suggest, to bacterial putrefaction; but in the absence of cultures it remains to be proved that the unruptured membranes are not an effectual barrier against the passage of bacteria from the vagina to the amniotic cavity.

Although under suitable conditions a great variety of pathologic bacteria may invade the amniotic fluid, the streptococcus has been the predominating organism found in cases of placental bacteremia. Frequently colon bacilli are associated with streptococci. In the case of tympanitis uteri during labor the colon bacillus was regarded as the exclusive etiologic factor until, in one instance, Krönig[5] demonstrated an obligatory anaerobic bacillus. Warnekros[6] has isolated the

4. Lehmann, Carpentier, Brieglet, Lendanthal, quoted by Hellendall, Note 3.
5. Krönig: Centralbl. f. Gynäk., 1894, xviii, 749; ibid., 1905, xxix, 1243.
6. Warnekros: Arch. f. Gynäk., 1913, c, 173.

gas bacillus from blood cultures in several cases of placental bacteremia. And in one of my cases placental sections showed a short, stout bacillus corresponding morphologically with the *Bacillus aerogenes capsulatus* though its identity was not established by means of cultures.

From the nature of the lesion in placental bacteremia, an infection within the uterus, generally limited to the amnion and the chorion and often most pronounced in the neighborhood of the large vessels passing over the fetal surface of the placenta, the associated clinical problem pertains both to the mother and to the child. Thus far, its maternal aspects have aroused the greatest interest. And this interest has been stimulated chiefly by a desire to determine whether a true uterine infection was responsible for intrapartum fever.

Glockner[7] thought the existence of an infection was unnecessary to explain intrapartum fever. Frequently in these cases the temperature becomes normal immediately after delivery, or presents only a slight temporary rise during the puerperium. Consequently, Glockner assumed pathogenic bacteria were not present, and ascribed the intrapartum symptoms to prolonged and violent uterine contractions. Winter[8] favored this view but also admitted that bacteria might be indirectly concerned. According to Winter's hypothesis the symptoms were occasionally explained by the absorption of toxins from a decomposing ovum. On the other hand, Hausen, Krönig, and Hellendall declared that intrapartum fever, like puerperal fever, depended on a bacterial invasion of the maternal tissues.

It occurred to Warnekros that this difference of opinion could be settled if cultures were made from the mother's blood in case her temperature during

---

7. Glockner: Ztschr. f. Geburtsh. u. Gynäk., 1891, xxi, 386.
8. Winter: Quoted by Meyer-Ruegg in Handb. d. Geburtshülfe, ii, Part 3, p. 2375.

labor rose above 38.5 C. The procedure was adopted in 25 cases; the cultures from 18 cases were positive, from 7, negative. In 9 instances streptococci were isolated, in 3 staphylococci, and in the other positive cases colon bacilli, pseudodiphtheria bacilli, or anaerobic gas-producing bacilli; not infrequently more than one type of organism was isolated. Whenever a positive culture was obtained during labor, another was made on the day following delivery. The puerperal cultures were negative except in one instance—the case of a patient who died of a streptococcus septicemia on the third day postpartum.

In approximately 70 per cent. of the cases of intrapartum fever it was clear that a genuine, if temporary, infection of the mother existed. The cause of the fever in the other cases was uncertain. Consequently, the scope of the investigation was broadened, and sections of the placenta were stained for bacteria. In every instance, even though the blood cultures had been negative, organisms were found in the placenta. And, therefore, Warnekros concluded that intrapartum fever, unless attributable to some accidental cause, as tuberculosis, was due to an infection of the mother, often mild and temporary, and that a placental bacteremia was always demonstrable.

The character of the puerperium which will follow a febrile labor may best be predicted from the result of blood cultures taken the day after delivery. Generally, these are negative and a good prognosis is assured. On the other hand, positive cultures indicate the existence of a puerperal infection. Blood cultures at the time of labor have no prognostic value. Similarly, as a prognostic sign the degree of fever at the time of labor is unreliable, for Winckel[9] observed several patients who experienced a puerperal convalescence free from fever in spite of an intrapartum temperature above 39 C. (102.2 F.).

9. Winckel: Quoted by Kronig, Note 5.

The puerperal morbidity in cases of intrapartum fever, an average based on the report of 944 cases by five observers, would seem to be about 63 per cent., the puerperal mortality 6.2 per cent.

RESULTS FOR THE MOTHER FOLLOWING
INTRAPARTUM FEVER

	No. of Cases	Normal Puerperium Per Cent.	Slight Fever Per Cent.	Severe Fever Per Cent.	No. of Deaths
Ahlfeld[1]	62	35.5	29.8	35.5	3
Glockner[2] ...	211	62.5	15.16	22.27	13
Ihm[3]	190	58.43	25.27	13.69	8
Kronig[4]	37	21.6	.....	78.4	7
Hellendall[5] ..	44	6.54	63.63	29.54	1

1. Ztschr. f. Geburtsh. u. Gynäk., 1893, xxvii, 494.
2. Ztschr. f. Geburtsh. u. Gynäk., 1891, xxi, 409.
3. Ztschr. f. Geburtsh. u. Gynäk., 1904, lii, p. 30.
4. Centralbl. f. Gynäk., 1894, xviii, 749; ibid., 1905, xxix, 1243.
5. Beitr. z. Geburtsh. u. Gynäk., 1906, x, 320.

In case of intrapartum fever the outlook is much more serious for the infant than for the mother. The fetal mortality encountered by Ihm was 18 per cent., by Hellendall 19 per cent., by Winter 35 per cent., and by Kronig 61 per cent. These statistics include cases of toxemia of pregnancy, of placenta praevia, of pelvic contraction, and of malposition of the fetus. Therefore, the death of the fetus may have been due to one of several causes, and, lacking the requisite examination, it is impossible to determine to what extent the infection of the placenta was concerned.

At present I am content to emphasize the fact that intrapartum infection must be regarded as one cause of fetal death, and also to demonstrate that the umbilical vessels may be the path of the infection. Heretofore, it has been assumed that antepartum infection of the fetus depended on its swallowing or aspirating the infected amniotic fluid. At most, Krönig has said, blood-borne infections to the fetus are limited to cases in which the mother is suffering from septicemia, as in typhoid fever, pneumonia, tuberculosis or cholera. But another possibility must be reckoned with, namely this: If the amniotic fluid is infected, the bacteria may cross the amnion and invade the placental vessels which carry blood to the fetus.

In one instance I have noted an intense infection of the subamniotic connective tissue and have demonstrated streptococci in the vessels on the fetal surface of the placenta and also in the umbilical vein. In another, streptococci were found in the placenta and in the cord, not in the lumen of the vein but in its wall. As further evidence that the cord infection proceeded from the placenta rather than the fetus no inflammatory lesion of the fetal respiratory or gastro-intestinal tract was found in any case. Various fetal organs were stained for bacteria but none were demonstrated.

It is also instructive that an examination of the placenta for bacteria occasionally serves to establish the cause of fetal death. Until this examination was made, the death of one infant which presented at necropsy a general peritonitis was attributed to imperfect nursery hygiene. Obviously, that explanation was excluded by the demonstration of streptococci in the placenta. Again, in the second case of placental bacteremia, the clinical diagnosis was hemophilia, and human blood serum was administered; the necropsy added nothing to the clinical findings. Also, in the third case the cause of the death of the fetus was not established clinically nor by postmortem; without appropriate study of the placenta the diagnosis could not have been made.

Placental bacteremia is not always attended by the death of the fetus or the newly born infant. This would not be expected. Bacterial invasion of the amnion and the chorion does not mean that the fetal blood vessels will necessarily become involved. The invasion may advance in another direction. Furthermore, the period of time elapsing between the invasion of the amnion and the birth of the infant may be too short for the organisms to reach the blood vessels in question. Clinical evidence corroborates this view; in cases of intrapartum fever, at most, two thirds of the infants perish.

This series of cases is not large enough to justify an uncompromising estimate of the part placental bacteremia plays in infant mortality. The fact, however, that three of twenty-seven deaths were attributable to this cause shows that it must be taken seriously into account. Perhaps it explains an appreciable number of the fetal and infant deaths heretofore impossible of explanation. Therefore, it is pertinent to recall the frequency of certain phenomena which are usually associated with bacterial invasion of the fetus.

Premature rupture of the membranes was noted by Bassett[10] five hundred times in 4,141 consecutive confinements and by Dmelin[11] four hundred times in 4,000 confinements. Thus, the frequency of this accident may be estimated to be between 10 and 15 per cent. On the other hand, Winckel and Krönig regard 3 per cent. as a fair estimate for the frequency of intrapartum fever. Basing a calculation on these statistics, it appears, if the membranes rupture prematurely, bacterial invasion of the placenta occurs in every fourth or fifth case. In view of these facts the routine study of the placenta for the purpose of demonstrating bacteria should be undertaken not only when the labor is febrile but also if it is prolonged after the membranes rupture.

150 York Street.

10. Bassett: Ztschr. f. Geburtsh. u. Gynäk., lxxiii, 566.
11. Dmelin: Quoted by Bassett, Note 10.

ABORTION

ITS CAUSES AND TREATMENT

E. E. MONTGOMERY, M.D., LL.D.

Fellow of the American College of Surgeons; Professor of Gynecology,
Jefferson Medical College

PHILADELPHIA

The present age is one of conservation. In every line of human industry the effort is made to preserve and utilize Nature's forces. In the machine shop and factory, careful study is made to prevent loss of material and energy. Fortunes are acquired through the utilization of by-products which formerly were allowed to waste. The great exception to this rule is in the promotion and preservation of the race. Every gynecologist who studies the histories of those who pass under his ministration must be impressed with the terrible sacrifice of human life, purposely or accidentally, during the period of gestation. The mental attitude of many individuals is such as to impress one that they regard the sole purpose of their union to be their personal gratification, rather than to propagate the race and preserve the species. Their study is how to gratify desire, and to avoid its consequences. Procreation, the higher purpose of such association, is regarded as an unfortunate sequel to be avoided if possible, or entertained only when the conditions may seem opportune. When such a mental attitude is assumed toward the processes of life, the disappointment is grievous when the exercise of the sexual function results in conception. Such persons are distressed by and offended at the physician who informs them there is no immune period or uninjurious means to prevent it. The couple who have

entered wedlock with the avowed determination to
avoid the discomforts and responsibilities incident to
pregnancy are mentally prepared to go further and
institute measures to arrest life's processes, and
destroy the life whose germination has been entrusted
to their fostering care. It is a sad reproach on our
civilization, an ominous danger to our nation, that
those who are able to and should find delight in rear-
ing and fostering their offspring will allow themselves
to be diverted therefrom by less weighty matters.
Our profession could not do a greater service to
humanity and to the state than to continually impress
on such patients the sanctity of human life in all its
processes, and that procreation is the primary purpose for mating of the sexes. We must admire and
respect those women who regard sterility as a
reproach, and loss of the immature embryo as a cause
for grief and distress.

Aside from any moral issue, Nature asserts her
penalty on all who violate her laws. Changes occur
in the genital structure of those who practice measures
to avoid conception, which render them subsequently
less prone to pregnancy, so that having reached a
period when they desire offspring their hopes are
denied. The changes are more marked in those who
have interrupted the course of gestation. The inflammatory processes resulting unfit the uterine mucosa
for the proper nourishment of its incumbent, and
abortion becomes a habit; a habit which is to be
overcome only by the restoration of affected structures
to a healthy condition. It is possible for inflammation
through infection to induce such injuries of the muscular structures of the uterus, tubes and pelvic peritoneum, as to render the uterus unable to enlarge
sufficiently to permit the maturing of the fetus; or
the tubes are so contracted that no opportunity is
afforded for the union of a spermatozoid with an
ovum, or the impregnated ovum is prevented from

entering the uterus and a misplaced pregnancy results, adding to the gravity of the condition.

No one can consider the immediate and remote possible infective changes following interference with gestation without realizing the baneful influence of infection on the health of the individual. Pathogenic conditions are engendered which may be slight and evanescent, or there may be structural changes which absolutely preclude future procreation and handicap the individual for life — may even cause death. Although procreation may be continued, is it not possible that slight changes in the structure may so limit the nutrition of the ovum as to impair its complete development and thus affect the future mental or physical course of the offspring, and even influence its progeny? A widespread disinclination to procreation must have its influence on the interests of the nation. A nation's strength is dependent on the moral' and physical courage of its men; hence, any cause which tends to limit procreation among the fit becomes a double crime, injurious to the public as well as to the individual.

Some members of the profession are advocating the legalization of abortion. Could any course be more disastrous! In all aggregations of population vice and crime are controlled through the force of public opinion. In every large city there are those who thrive as professional abortionists, who are so protected by the sympathizers with vice as to make their conviction and punishment difficult. That the production of abortion is a crime, and its practice disreputable, deters the physician who has any regard for his reputation from its employment. Its legalization, however, opens a door for its more general practice, when patient and physician could regard such a course justified by law and within the choice of the affected individual. Such a situation becomes an encouragement to vice and immorality, and prejudicial to the interests of the state. Without question every physician is familiar with unfortunate instances when girls of good family have been victimized or have yielded to overpowering temptation, but these do not justify interference with the laws of life by arresting its progress. However much the social situation of such individuals and their parents appeals to the physician, it should be an accepted dogma that those who violate the laws of society must pay the penalty.

CAUSES

Abortion may be the result of overexertion, infection or injury, but most frequently in first pregnancies through efforts to secure evacuation of the uterine contents by the administration of drugs or by mechanical measures. When the uterus is the seat of disease from previous infection or interruption of pregnancy, the pathogenic changes render the organ incapable of nourishing the incumbent until full term, and the contents are evacuated. When pregnancy recurs abortion becomes a habit. Frequently this is attributed to syphilis, which may be the cause, but it occurs more frequently independent of it.

TREATMENT

The treatment of abortion consists in the preventive when threatened; the prophylactic when conditions exist which ensure its occurrence or when pregnancy occurs in cases in which the tendency has become a habit; and finally, completion of the evacuation of the uterus when abortion is inevitable, or has partially occurred.

Threatened abortion is best treated by absolute rest. The exclusion of all causes of excitement, the administration of an opiate, preferably by suppository or hypodermically, an easily digested, nutritious diet, the administration of laxatives and avoidance of remedies such as ergot, cotton root, quinin and strychnin, which increase the uterine irritability.

The prophylactic treatment is employed with those who have previously aborted, while nonpregnant, and consists in the improvement of the pelvic condition. The use of the curet in endometritis; surgical treatment of lacerations, extensive abrasions, eversion of the mucosa and extensive involvement of the racemose glands of the cervix should be regarded as indicated. Retrodisplacements and prolapsus should be corrected. A syphilitic history should be an indication for antisyphilitic treatment, and in all cases of habitual abortion, whether specific or nonspecific, potassium iodid will be found an invaluable agent. Its administration should not only precede pregnancy, but should be continued with more or less persistency during the early months. This drug diminishes the irritability of the uterine mucosa and ensures the continuance of pregnancy when an abortion would otherwise be inevitable.

INEVITABLE AND INCOMPLETE ABORTION

When it becomes evident that abortion will occur in spite of measures to avoid it, the early aseptic evacuation of the uterus is advisable. The natural inclination of the physician when consulted by a patient who has undergone a recent abortion is to make sure that the embryonic products have been completely evacuated, particularly if there are present symptoms of infection as indicated by elevation of temperature, rapid pulse, tenderness over the abdomen and pain in the pelvis. The friends of the patient attribute such phenomena to retention of portions of the products of gestation, and are insistent on measures for removal. When the symptoms are not ameliorated they become obsessed with the idea that the procedure has not been complete, and in many instances secure another consultant to repeat the process. No plan of treatment could be more detrimental to the interests of the patient.

During the five years, inclusive from 1910 to 1914, there have been treated in the gynecologic wards at

Jefferson Hospital, 296 patients who were admitted under the designation of incomplete abortion. The great majority of these patients were suffering from symptoms of infection on admission; in many of them infection was well advanced and the condition practically hopeless. Many of them had undergone curettement prior to entering the hospital; 127, or nearly 43 per cent., were subjected to some surgical procedure after admission. There were 13 deaths in the entire number admitted; 5 of these were subjected to surgical measures after admission, while 8 were not treated surgically. The apparent percentage of mortality is 3.8 per cent. for those surgically treated, and 4.7 for the medically treated cases. At first glance it would appear that surgical measures afforded the most hope, but it must be remembered that no patients were refused admission, and only those were subjected to surgical procedures in whom local foci of infection were evident. While the profoundly infected patients were treated by supportive measures, careful analysis of the cases convinces me that a smaller mortality would have occurred had we received these patients before they had been subjected to any surgical interference, and subsequently confined our treatment to nonsurgical measures.

Nature has arranged her forces to expel the uterine contents when they have completed their function, or when they are no longer in condition to continue it. In addition she affords ample protection against infection unless her barriers are injudiciously broken down. Every examination and all manipulation of the genital structures of an aborting patient should be strictly aseptic, and when such conditions are difficult to attain, the vulva should be kept covered with clean napkins wrung out of a mixture of equal quantities of alcohol and water, while pituitary extract should be administered hyopdermically to promote expulsion of contents and closure of vessels.

It is often hard to resist one's inclination, and the importunities of relatives of the infected individual that some interference should be made in patients appearing with symptoms of infection following abortion, but it should be remembered that even admitting the retention of embryonic products, the infective organisms to not limit themselves to the local area. If they have not already invaded the blood, the manipulation necessary to explore and remove the retained tissue breaks down the barriers Nature has erected against further invasion.

1426 Spruce Street.

ABSTRACT OF DISCUSSION

DR. ALFRED BAKER SPALDING, San Francisco: Retroversion of the uterus predisposes to abortion in the early stages of pregnancy probably more than any other one thing, and often causes the death of the fetus; the so-called "blighted ovum." The attendant who corrects the retroversion is often unjustly blamed for the death or miscarriage of the fetus. I have in my laboratory several specimens of blighted ovum passed some months after replacement of a pregnant retroverted uterus which show an early stage of development at the time of death.

There has been for some years a growing tendency among gynecologists and men of experience to present to the profession the idea that the surgical emptying of the uterus is bad in principle and bad in practice. I am not one who agrees with this statement. There is undoubtedly a difference between the infected and the uninfected patient following the abortion; but in either case it has been my practice, and the practice of Dr. Somers, who preceded me in the woman's clinic of Stanford University, to dilate and curet the uterus immediately after the patient enters the hospital. I do not know what Dr. Somers' results have been, but I do know my experience. In the last three years we have had eighty-six patients enter with symptoms of incomplete abortion. All, with the exception of one, were treated surgically. One was not treated. Three were treated by means of manual curettement of the uterus and the other eighty-two patients were treated by dilatation and curettage. None of these patients had been curetted before entering the hospital, which may make a difference in the statistics. Of these eighty-six patients only one died. Dr. Stephenson gathered together as many of these histories as possible. Of the forty patients reviewed, the temperature was normal on admission to the hospital in thirteen cases and from 99 to 103 in twenty-seven cases. After operation, the temperature either remained normal from the day of operation or returned to normal in seventeen cases; ten were normal the first day after operation, making twenty-seven cases; five returned to normal on the second day after operation, making thirty-two; three returned to normal on the third day, making thirty-five; one returned to normal on the fourth day, making thirty-six; two, fifth day following operation, making thirty-eight, while only two persisted with elevated temperature for seven days. Twenty-three had a leukocytosis before operation of over 9,000, some as high as 30,000, showing another evidence of probable infection. As to the cause, twenty-four stated that abortion came on spontaneously, and sixteen acknowledged that they had brought it on criminally. Of late it has been our practice to test the mothers for syphilis in case of an unexplained abortion. In four recent cases, all gave a negative Wassermann on examination. I present these statistics, hurriedly gathered together, to show that patients can be well treated by clearing out the uterus promptly, although at the same time I am sure Dr. Montgomery can in general practice show that many patients can empty the uterus spontaneously and are better untampered with. I wish to point out, however, that at present I cannot see the reason for not emptying the uterus in abortion.

DR. JOHN OSBORN POLAK, Brooklyn: Before this section and before the American Gynecological Society we have called attention for several years to the treatment of infected cases by the so-called palliative methods (so-called judicious neglect plan) versus operative procedure, and our results have been so exceptionally good that we have rather felt that the profession should share with us in the little knowledge that we have gained by the study of this procedure.

We divide abortions into the infected and the noninfected cases. I do not believe that any of us feel that in a noninfected case the uterus cannot be entered with safety and if the evacuation is complete and clear, perhaps the convalescence of that patient will be expedited; but I do know that the infected case which has protected itself, as each infected case does protect itself, by a leukocytic wall, and if a placenta is present and thrombi are formed in the vessels in the placenta site, that the infection is spread and the patient's condition is jeopardized by the routine procedure of curettage.

The question of interference in abortion is this: Is there hemorrhage or is there not hemorrhage? If there is no hemorrhage, our experience has been, even when the temperature is 104 or 105, that those patients, if placed in the Fowler position, an ice pack put over the abdomen and elimination maintained with saline solution and intestinal rest, with no cathartics and no food, show—inside of twenty-four to seventy-two hours—great improvement; the products will separate, for they have been starved off by the formation of the round-cell deposits, and the product of conception will be delivered completely, if left alone, in the large majority of cases. If it is not delivered spontaneously, it is found with the uterus contracted and this large mass lying in the dilated lower segment of the uterus. We have, for instance, reported twenty consecutive infected cases, before the International Congress, with the complete contents of conception left *in situ*; every one of those patients made a complete recovery, the uterus expelling its contents spontaneously, and we believe just in proportion as these cases are interefered with, so is the morbility increased. In a hundred consecutive cases, sixty-three had been curetted one or more times, and all of these showed exudates. On the other hand, in 200 consecutive cases admittedly infected, without interference, we found that in this series of cases our morbidity as to exudates and as to mortality was decreased. It is a pleasure to hear Dr. Montgomery, whose word covers such weight, protest against this active interference in abortion.

Dr. C. Lester Hall, Kansas City, Mo.: We all feel keenly the outrage that has been committed by the profession on the pregnant woman in the way of producing abortion. It is now many years since I first heard a man, or several men of high standing, in the discussion of this subject, flatly acknowledge a willingness to produce abortion in the maiden who had been unfortunately caught. My protest on that occasion, whether it had any lasting effects or not, was so emphatic that it has been my good fortune not to hear these men repeat this statement. The outrage is so monstrous that we cannot accentuate it too strongly. I feel that it is not done now as it once was done. I believe the profession is rising above this nefarious practice. In regard to the treatment of abortions, I think it depends very much on circumstances. I believe it would be justifiable in almost any case, if the obstetrician were sufficiently clean, to empty the uterus with a blunt instrument; to swab out the uterus once, and never again. It is the continual meddling that brings dire results, and even with all our care it is liable to produce septic conditions.

I know the value of the protective wall that nature has thrown out, and over and over again it has been my fortune, and I believe with good results, to stay the hand of the energetic, aspiring young obstetrician who wanted continually to meddle with these cases. We know the deleterious effect of uterine douching. In regard to giving these patients potassium iodid, that Dr. Montgomery refers to, to make a woman carry a baby to term, I would object to the giving of the potash. I think we might give iodin itself with safety, but in all these cases we are apt to have more or less kidney trouble, and I believe in giving potassium iodid we load up the system with this potash which is toxic and detrimental. I protest that in women with albuminuric conditions we should avoid the use of potassium iodid or other potash salts.

In regard to retrodisplacements of the uterus of the pregnant woman, it is a great misfortune if we cannot institute some measure whereby we can make this woman carry her child to term and prevent the recurrence of the retrodisplacements. This is the *only* nonsurgical way we can correct these displacements. This I have often done, and by the postural treatment after delivery recurrence of the retrodisplacement has been prevented. This will happen in 99 per cent. of all cases in which the retrodisplacement has existed before pregnancy.

The subject is so important, and coming from Dr. Montgomery, is so effective that I am sure if any young man here has been imprudent in the use of instruments after abortions, the doctor's paper will have a lasting good effect, and it will do us *all* a great deal of good.

Dr. S. M. D. Clark, New Orleans: It seems that we are about to agree on some standard method in handling abortions. In noninfected cases I believe with Dr. Montgomery the sanest plan is to empty the uterus with as little traumatism as possible and then leave an iodin wick for twenty four hours. The infected abortions are the ones on which there are still divergent opinions. It took a goodly experience before I could break away from the old plan of emptying the uterus in these cases. After all, the pathology should guide us, and when this is thoroughly understood, the locally inactive plan is the method that best complies with these laws. When called in consultation, how often have each of us found the physician giving daily intrauterine douches; he generally curets and if the temperature materially rises, feeling that there is still something remaining, he again curets. The pressure of the anxious family forces him into some local activity; he feels that he must be doing something, so he goes ahead douching and curetting. This daily mauling is repeated, not so much for the patient, but for the family. Where the infection is already beyond the endometrium, nothing could be more unreasonable than to expect relief by superficially fussing around in the interior of the uterus. Let such cases alone, adopt the locally inactive plan, furnish an abundance of fluids and keep the patients well nourished. The infection in practically every case will localize; an immunity will be established; the patient will autogenously vaccinate herself and the exudate either resolve or suppurate.

The importance of the lower segment of the uterus in these infected abortion cases has not been given due consideration. In many of our cases the upper segment is never involved, but rather the infection has struck directly out toward the parametrium through the richly supplied lymphatic circulation of the cervix. This is the type in which the true pelvic connective tissue abscess is found, which when drained is immediately cured. Could anything be more unreasonable than to curet in such cases? I think a point to be driven home is the extreme importance of exercising the most rigid asepsis when making vaginal examinations in diagnosing cases of abortion. The vaginal canal should be explored with the same aseptic regard as one would invade a knee joint or the abdominal cavity.

Dr. H. G. Wetherill, Denver: In the treatment of these cases it is important to determine whether one is dealing with a spontaneous abortion or a mechanically induced abortion. Infections of the genital tract are commonly retrograde infections if the abortion is mechanically induced, or if there has been gynecologic tinkering. If, on the other hand, it is an incomplete abortion, not of the mechanical type, then we certainly are justified in picking out with the placental forceps any retained portion of the product of conception which might otherwise give rise to sapremia. With this exception, I agree wholly with the principles of treatment set forth by Dr. Montgomery and I am heartily in accord with him in his strictures on the abuse of the uterine curet in such cases. So careful should we be in handling infected cases that a tenaculum or volsellum forceps should not be used to draw down and fix the cervix, as the small punctures made by the teeth of the instrument are sufficient to reinoculate a patient from the vaginal and cervical secretion.

For many years I have treated infections following abortions with alcohol after the method of Caruso. A double drainage tube of large caliber is inverted on itself, so that the solution cannot follow the tube. This tube is introduced to the fundus with strict antiseptic precautions and the alcohol which is used through it flushes the genital tract from the fundus outward with a nonpoisonous, antiseptic solution. Occasionally a solution of permanganate of potash or a diluted solution of iodin is substituted for the alcohol. In the treatment of such cases it is very easy to do too much and almost impossible to do too little. The majority of the patients will recover if let alone.

Dr. E. E. Montgomery, Philadelphia: I must confess that if called to a woman who had an abortion or was aborting, in whom a portion of the embryo had escaped, whom I had reason to feel was not an infected case, and in making a careful aseptic examination discovered a portion of the placenta projecting, I should be tempted at once to evacuate the uterus; but in cases such as one of the gentlemen mentioned in which the mass is situated within the body of the organ, the cervix, possibly, more or less contracted, the result of leaving the case to nature, treating it carefully, aseptically, will be attended with much less danger to the patient than would be the mechanical dilatation of the uterus and the removal of the structures within. I believe, also, in those cases of which Dr. Wetherill has spoken, in which a portion of the placenta remains and it is evident that sapremia exists, it is better to leave the condition undisturbed and trust nature to evacuate it rather than use mechanical measures.

THE HISTOGENESIS OF THE REPRODUCTIVE PROCESSES IN MAMMALS

HENRY O. MARCY, A.M., M.D., LL.D.

BOSTON

One of the most interesting questions presenting itself to the investigator, and which has been surrounded with the deepest mystery, is that of the vital processes of the reproduction of animal life. From the earliest periods of medicine may be traced the results of observation and the deductions therefrom which have given rise to speculative theories and beliefs.

Fabricius[1] made careful studies of the placenta. He demonstrated that the placenta varied in position, shape, and size in mammals, laying emphasis on the form of a placenta found in the human animal. He concluded that the single placenta found in the human female, the mouse, the rabbit, the guinea-pig, the dog and the cat, is associated with the presence of incisor teeth in both jaws and with distinct toes. When the placenta is found multiple, as in the sheep, the cow, and goat the incisors are present in one jaw only, and the hoofs are cloven.

Malpighi[2] was among the first to make careful scientific studies of the changes which take place in the uterus and the developing ovum. The microscope had become an instrument of value. Histologic changes were traced by him with a skill worthy of the great master which he was. His name is deservedly prominent on the roll of the famous teachers and investi-

---

1. Fabricius: De Formato Foetu, 1624, Folio.
2. Malpighi, Marcello: Born in 1628, died in 1694; he was Professor of the University of Bologna about twenty-five years. He was appointed physician to Pope Innocent XII, and for some years lived in Rome.

gators of his period. He is entitled to the appellation
of "The Founder of Microscopic Anatomy." His
study of the secretory glands and their structures led
to the inference that the secretion is formed in terminal acini, standing in open connection with the ducts.

William Hunter of London[3] studied the early development of the placenta of woman with extreme care
and his beautifully illustrated folio volume will ever
remain a classic of English medical literature.

William Hunter's work on the reproductiveness of
woman must remain of permanent value. In Plate 32,
Figure 36, he gives a careful drawing of the decidua
vera of the fifth week of pregnancy.

> It plainly appears that the decidua in this case was a thick
> membrane of gelatinous texture, which had lived and adhered
> to the whole triangular cavity of the fundus uteri; that the
> tubes terminated on its internal surface; that the chorion
> was lodged in its duplicature, or was surrounded with its
> substance; and that in the proportion as the chorion would
> have been extended in the progress of gestation, it would
> have encroached on the cavity of the decidua, stretching its
> interior lamella or decidua reflexa, till at length, the cavity
> being obliterated, that interior lamella would have come into
> contact with the inside of the decidua.

He describes an abortion at the ninth week when the
embryo hangs by a slender navel string from the inside
of the placenta. The amnion, the chorion, and the
decidua reflexa are adherent to one another. Here
the larger and more crowded branches of the shaggy
vessels which shoot from the external surface of one
part of the chorion mix with the decidua, or uterine
part, to form the placenta.

Here is seen a portion of a chorion which afterwards
becomes the uniform transparent membrane. It is
covered with fewer and more delicate floating vessels,
which lose themselves in the decidua reflexa. The
embryo is seen through it.

Montgomery of Dublin published a most interesting
book on human gestation, emphasizing a discovery of

---

3. Hunter, William: Anatomia Uteri Humani Gravidi.

his own, made and published four or five years previous, of a peculiarity in the structure of the decidua vera.

If the ovum is expelled entire, we have the uterine decidua covering the substance under examination and distinguished by its soft, rich, pulpy appearance and strong red color; its external or uterine surface being rough and unequal and when well freed from the coagulated blood and immersed in water, exhibiting numerous small round foramina, capable of admitting the head of a pin; while its internal surface is smooth, generally thrown into slight, soft folds, and exhibits little or no appearance of foramina; any that may be perceptible being of very minute size. These characters, which are always to be recognized without difficulty, are sufficiently distinctive of the structure under consideration; but there is another, not hitherto noticed by anyone as far as I am aware, although it is probably one of the most remarkable features in the organization of this peculiar product. Repeated examinations have shown me that there are, on the external surface of the decidua vera, a great number of small cup-like elevations, having the appearance of little bags, the bottoms of which are attached to, or embedded in, its substance; they then expand or belly out a little, and again grow smaller towards their outer or uterine end which in by far the greater number of them, is an open mouth when separated from the uterus; how it may be while they are adherent I cannot at the present say. Some of them which I have found more deeply embedded in the decidua vera are completely closed sacs. Their form is circular, or very nearly so; they vary in diameter from a twelfth to a sixth of an inch, and project about a twelfth of an inch from the surface of the decidua. Altogether they give one the idea of miniature representations of the suckers of the cuttle-fish. They are not confined to any part of the surface of the decidua, but I think I have generally found them most numerous and distinct on those parts of it which were not connected with the capillary rudiments of a placenta, and at the period of gestation which precedes the formation of the latter as a distinct organ. They are best seen about the second or third month and they are not to be found at the advance periods of gestation. I confess that I am not prepared (nor indeed is this the place) to offer any very decided opinion as to the precise nature or use of these decidual cotyledons, for to that name their form, as well as their situation, appears strictly to entitle them; but from having on more than one occasion observed within their cavity a milky or chylous fluid, I am disposed to consider them reservoirs for nutriment fluids separated from the maternal blood, to be thence absorbed for the support and development of the ovum. This view seems strengthened when we consider that at the early periods of gestation the ovum derives all its support by imbibition through the connection existing between the decidua and the villous processes covering the outer surface of the chorion.[4]

Prof. Charles S. Minot, in his "Theory of the Placenta," says:

According to the views explained in the preceding pages, I hold the placenta to be an organ of the chorion; that primitively the chorion had its own circulation, and formed the discoidal placenta by developing villi, which grew down into the degenerating uterine mucosa. By the degeneration of the maternal tissues, the maternal blood is brought close to the villi, and the degeneration may go so far that all the tissue of the uterus between the villi and the muscularis uteri go to form the so-called decidua; the placenta receives its fetal blood by the means of large vessels running in the mesoderm of the allantois. From this discoidal chorionic placenta, the zonary placenta of carnivora, the diffuse placenta of the lower primates, and the metadiscoidal placenta of woman, have been evolved.

Dr. Minot was a man of erudition and enthusiastically devoted to science. By his recent death Harvard University has lost one of her famous pupils and distinguished teachers. His postgraduate education was in Germany, and to the last he adopted as correct the conclusions of the German school. All this I accepted as fundamentally correct until I became acquainted with the researches of Ercolani, professor in the great University of Bologna. I found by accident in a second-hand book store in Paris a very cheaply printed unpretentious volume published in Algiers, Africa, a translation in French by Dr. Andreni, of a certain portion of the investigations which had been conducted by Professor Ercolani. As a prize essay it had received an award from the Academy of Science at Paris.

Ercolani was a count, and cousin of the present king of Italy; like my old master, Professor Virchow of Berlin, he was equally celebrated as a leader in the

---

4. Montgomery, W. F.: Signs and Symptoms of Pregnancy, London, 1837.

great political struggles for the elevation of his people, and as an enthusiastic devotee of science educated in the schools of the great Antonio Alessandrini, whose diligence the pupil early imitated. Under the most lamentable poverty of means, he contributed to the foundation of those monuments of marvelous industry, the Bologna museums of comparative anatomy and veterinary pathologic anatomy.

The high renown which Ercolani had acquired in the sciences, together with his profound learning, procured for him many honors. He attained the highest offices of Bologna's most famous university, in which he was several times president of the medical faculty and twice rector of the university. Aided by government, he was enabled to erect new buildings and furnish the school of veterinary medicine with modern appliances for successfully carrying on original investigations in the department of comparative anatomy and physiology. Although widely known by his many original contributions to science, he is deserving of, and he receives, world-wide repute for his long-continued investigations of the placental development in vertebrates.

In our Harvard library, I found in the Bologna Transactions of the Academy of Sciences the original papers, with illustrations, published from time to time, having been presented by him as contributions to the academy. Convinced of the singular value, as well as the originality of his work, I collated and presented to the English reading public my first edition, which included all his anatomic researches up to the date of the publication. The closing chapters were written especially for this American edition. In 1884 I published a second and enlarged edition, which included also Professor Ercolani's researches on the pathologic conditions of placental development, with a careful analytic review of the whole subject, written while yet suffering from the dire malady which speedily thereafter terminated his life.

In the preface to the second edition of my translation of Ercolani's work I say:

I have myself confirmed many of the observations of the learned author and I have therefore repeated assurance of the correctness of his statements and deductions. As if, with the foreknowledge of his untimely end, immediately before his death, Prof. Ercolani reviewed his entire work in extenso with a long résumé of his carefully established conclusions. This summary is also included in the present volumes. I am convinced of the correctness of Prof. Ercolani's teaching. I hold in admiration the remarkable ability and certainty by which he arrived at conclusions so far-reaching and demonstrated with singular clearness nature's uniform law of the unity of anatomic type in a simple and fundamental plan of embryonic nutrition and development.

The present occasion offers an opportunity to review very briefly some of the more important deductions to be made therefrom. The studies of reproduction by the medical profession have been chiefly limited to the human species. Nothing is more complex or confusing, more a veritable labyrinthine riddle,[5] than the fully developed human placenta.[6]

There are many and varying factors which must be taken into careful consideration in the study of the miracle of reproduction. Many of these must necessarily be eliminated from this article. First and most important is the matured ovum, which is usually impregnated in the fallopian tube. The cellular segmentation which goes on in the first days; the implantation of the ovum and its subsequent development, is a chapter foreign to the histogenesis of uterine life in the present discussion, except so far as pertains to the nutrition and growth of the fetus. Even here, we must limit ourselves for the most part to the early histologic changes which occur in the fetal structures.

The two important series of structures presenting themselves for investigation in the anatomy of the placenta are the fetal villi, of the chorion and the

5. The deductions of the earlier writers were clothed in fable quite as much as the Golden Fleece.

6. Ercolani, Giovanni Battista: The Reproductive Process — Its Histology, Physiology and Pathology, Demonstrating the Unity of the Anatomical Type of the Placenta in all the Mammalia and the Physiological Unity of the Nutrition of the Foetus in all the Vertebrates. Translated by Henry O. Marcy, A.M., M.D., Boston, Houghton, Mifflin & Co., Riverside Press, 1884.

maternal villi. These component parts form the placenta. The complexity of its structure in any given mammal is dependent on the degree to which, in the course of its development and growth, the maternal and the fetal portions have become interblended.

In the study of the reproductive processes of woman, these changes early become so complex that, except in the first weeks of pregnancy, very few definite conclusions can be drawn. The study of the changes taking place in the lower animals has been of the highest value. To William Turner of Edinburgh,[7] and G. V. Ercolani of Bologna, Italy, two of the most distinguished scientists of comparative anatomy, we are chiefly indebted for the elucidation of this problem. Turner arrived at the conclusion that the utricular glands are secreting structures, that they enlarge during pregnancy, and that their secretion is poured out between the mucous membrane and the chorion.

The demonstration seems complete that the main factor in the nutrition of the entire mammalian family, reduced to its simplest terms, is—a villus of secretion, maternal, and a villus of absorption, fetal. The maternal villi have their origin in the utricular glands, which are active during the entire reproductive period of the female.

These glands take on a singular activity at the so-called period of heat in the lower animals and about the period of menstruation in woman. In woman, these glands greatly enlarge and a proliferated portion breaks down in the processes of menstruation, quite to their base.

This disintegration goes on during the entire period of uterine activity. It may be playfully designated as "cleaning house" for the tenant which may never take possession, regardless of the sign "to let."

In extra-uterine fetation in woman, remarkable changes take place in the uterus proper, especially in

7. Turner, William: Lectures on the Comparative Anatomy of the Placenta, Edinburgh, 1876.

its inner coats. Here the glands, instead of undergoing the destructive processes of menstruation, take on a change not very unlike the first processes of impregnation. In some instances a veritable decidua is formed and the thickened velvety structure of the mucous membrane, with a greatly increased vascularity, is seldom wanting.

These maternal changes are instructive in their bearing on the development of the decidua vera in woman. In the first stages of uterine development, the chorion, which is the most external of the fetal membranes, is uniformly covered with delicate, slender villi of a soft, velvety appearance.

It is common knowledge that in woman the chorial villi in the early stage of development pertain almost uniformly to its entire surface and are at first interblended with the entire decidua vera. Later on, absorption takes place and these nearly disappear, leaving a translucent membrane except at, or near, the placental site. Then most complex changes take place, the chorial and the maternal villi interblending in the most confusing manner.

In the mare is found one of the simpler forms of placental development. The chorial villi persist during the entire period of gestation, for the most part uniformly developed, and here we find the intradigitation of the chorial and the placental villi comparatively easy for study, giving us perhaps the best demonstration of the simple plan of fetal nutrition — a villus of secretion in close approximation to, and blended with, a villus of absorption.

It is of extreme scientific interest to trace the multiple variations in the entire group of the mammalia. To this subject, however, we can only allude. In the ruminants, the villi are collected in large tufts called cotyledons, scattered over the surface of the chorion in very considerable numbers. In the cow, in one instance, I think I observed about eighty of them scattered uniformly over the entire chorion. These villi soon assume a complex form, budding from the side and end, and frequently assume an arborescent shape. The primal villus is the stem and the offshoots form the branches; these last are highly vascular.

The epithelial lining of the mucous membrane of the uterus is columnar in form in nearly all mammals. The utricular glands may be described as branching tubes which vary in length and direction in different mammals. My old friend Dr. G. J. Englemann of St. Louis[8] determined that no glands exist in the human uterus at birth. At the tenth year he found the glands assuming a tubular shape, becoming numerous and extending through the thickness of the mucosa into the muscular coat. Only at puberty do they become well developed and of active function.

Harvey[9] maintained that the fluid secreted by the cotyledons was absorbed by the fetal villi. Needham, of London,[10] yet more clearly insisted on the fact that the cotyledons were in function only secreting, while Haller[11] expressed the thought in a single sentence so terse that we quote: "In ruminantibus manifestam fit, matrem inter et foetum, non sanguinis sed lactis esse commerciam."

Analysis of this fluid by N. Gamgee[12] shows that it is alkaline, and contains besides water, albumin, fat and inorganic salts. A long known and well-established fact is that rudimentary cotyledons are never wanting in the nonpregnant state, but it remained for Ercolani to demonstrate that on the site was developed a new organ of glandular character and that it differed from the diffuse placenta chiefly in being developed over circumscribed areas and possessing a more complex character.

---

8. Englemann, G. J.: Am. Jour. Obst., May, 1875, p. 32.
9. Harvey: Opera Omnia, Leyden, 1737.
10. Needham: Padua, 1656.
11. Haller, London, 1767.
12. Gamgee, N.: Vet. Rev., No. 46, Edinburgh, 1864.

The single placenta, whether zonarial or discoidal, offers difficulties far greater to its satisfactory study because of its complexity of formation.

The bibliography of the subject forms a chapter in the literature of anatomy and physiology of exceptional interest to the special student, although most confusing to the seeker after knowledge. An admirable sketch of the observations made in this field of inquiry is found in the work of Ercolani above referred to.

We select for careful examination the gravid uterus of the rabbit. A transverse section of the placental site in the earlier period of pregnancy, about the end of the second week, shows three parts, each clearly distinct.

(1) The muscular wall of the uterus.

(2) The placental neoplasm which is developed on the inner uterine surface.

(3) Above this the old uterine mucous membranes tumefied and about to undergo destructive changes.

Two most noteworthy conditions appear. The uteroplacental vessels have a lumen almost double the vessels from which they proceed, and, notwithstanding their greater volume, they show in their walls none of the anatomic characteristics which serve to distinguish the arteries from the veins, and which are clearly visible in the uterine vessels. The second and even more important fact is that these vessels, instead of the ordinary walls, are surrounded with a uniform envelope of cells of a special character, which cannot be distinguished from the cells of the decidua serotina and the maternal placental tissue. The special characteristics of the walls of the vessels, composed, as they are seen to be, of only the endothelium, is an objection to the supposition that their development could proceed from the vascular net-work of the old transformed mucous membrane. This is emphasized by the exceptional fact that the old uterine mucous membrane is detached from the muscular wall, and, with its glands, is undergoing a process of rapid destruction. These facts place it beyond all doubt that the uteroplacental vessels and their surrounding cells are the result of a real neoformative process. In all animals having a single placenta the decidua vera and the decidua reflexa are of new and distinct formative character. The decidua vera is composed of newly formed cells, which are early arrested in their development, and superimposed on it is the old uterine mucous membrane, usually easily distingunished by its glands, and which, later, is seen in process of destruction and interblending between the external layer of the ovum and the internal uterine wall.

In most animals the newly formed placental vessels have a uniform diameter and constitute a network of small meshes, which reaches as far as, and is firmly joined to, the chorion. In the meshes of this network are found the fetal vessels which unite and enter the cord. By injection of these we have a better demonstration of the relations established between the fetal and maternal portion of the placenta. A careful study affords convincing proof that the umbilical arteries ramify and end in a thin, fine network of capillaries in the chorial villi, and are in close contact with the cellular covering which clothes the maternal vessels. Demonstrative evidence of this relationship in the human placenta has been frequently observed by myself when the placenta has been undisturbed in its connections with the uterus for a considerable period after the death of the fetus. The chorial villi become shrunken and easily separate from the decidual sheath, the cells of which remain unchanged.

In certain of the lower animals (for example, the *Cavia cobaya* or guinea-pig) Ercolani has observed that the maternal vessels become dilated in their terminal loops. This is of the greatest importance, since it furnishes an example in rudimentary condition of that which takes place in an extreme degree in the human placenta.

The destructive changes in the uterine mucous membrane of woman after conception are limited to the epithelial layer. After the separation of the decidua vera from the internal uterine surface, it is observed that the muscular wall is covered by a mucous membrane identical with that lining the uterine cavity before impregnation. The uterine mucous membrane is little more than a simple layer of epithelium, and the reproduction of this is all that is required to restore the internal surface of the uterus to its primary state.

During the early period of development of the human placenta the decidual cells form a richly vascular compact layer surrounding the chorial villi. For a limited time the relationship between the parts is not so intimate that they cannot be separated. At this stage, before the maternal vessels become ectasic, the form of development is not unlike the diffused or disseminated placenta.

Charles Robin states that in proportion as the villi of the chorion subdivide and increase in volume the superficial capillaries of the maternal placenta are largely dilated and form delicate vascular folds, which are interposed between them. The dilatations of the interposed maternal capillaries increase in direct ratio to the development of the chorial villi.

The walls of the proliferating branches of the villi are necessarily forced against the decidual layer of cells covering the ectasic thin-walled maternal vessel. Thus this is introflected, and a close union ensues. In this manner the so-called placental lacunae are formed in the fully developed placenta, and from this very deceptive appearance it has been held as a demonstrated fact that the fetal villi swim in the maternal blood.

Dr. John Reid was among the first to enunciate the belief that the fetal villi, in projecting, push before them the membranes forming the limiting wall of the placental sinuses, each of them in this way receiving an investment. Schroder van der Kolk and Goodsir taught that the processes of the decidua were prolonged over each villus, and thus separated it from the maternal sinus.

Braxton Hicks states that the placental sinuses, as usually represented, do not exist. He thinks the changes in the fetal blood are effected by endosmosis, but suggests that the follicles of the decidua may secrete a fluid which is poured into the intervillous spaces for absorption by the villi.

The epithelial covering of the vascular loop of the fetal villus is wanting because of the intimate relation which has been established between it and the secretory villus, which never loses its own epithelium. The form of the vascular loop of the maternal villus varies very greatly. In the quadrumana and in woman the dilatations become lacunose and are actually enormous.

All the vertebrates during the period of embryonic life, in order to complete the marvellous phases of their development, require a special nourishment, which is always furnished them by the mother. This is conveyed to and converted into its own substance by the embryo, and however many and considerable may be the differences met in these two fundamental factors, the unity running through them readily appears under two general forms, represented by the yolk of the egg in the oviparous animals and by the placenta in vertebrate mammals. In the first the maternal element is stored up in a mass by the mother, and emitted with the ovum in the quantity needed by the embryo to complete its development. In the second this nutritive material is furnished by the mother from the placenta, which elaborates it as needful for the developing embryo. These materials, in every case, are absorbed and conveyed to the fetus by means of its own vascular appendages. Thus nutrition is carried on during the development period in all vertebrates by a single law of physiologic modality. The typical anatomic form in the two fundamental parts of the placenta, however wide the variation, is always identical. It consists of a villus of new formation, maternal as well as fetal, each composed of an internal vascular loop surrounded by a cellular layer and covered by an outer epithelium. The office only of the villi is different—the fetal absorptive, the maternal secretive. These villi always come in contact more or less intimate, but the walls of the vascular loops never in any instance touch. This is the more to be emphasized since it invalidates the idea hitherto held, and yet almost universally taught, that the mode of the nutrition of the fetus is an interchange between the two bloods by endosmosis and exosmosis. The different ways of the interblending of the fetal and maternal villi give the complex and confusing picture of placental formation.

The belief that the lacunae were really large cavities as they certainly appeared, and not the maternal vessels greatly dilated, was held as a truth proved and indisputable; and it was through this belief that two other deceptive appearances were received as actual truths; namely, that the villi floated in the maternal blood, and that the epithelium covering them appertained to the fetus instead of to the mother.

This is another demonstration of science, showing that the great fundamental plan and law, in the last analysis, is based on pure and simple truth.

180 Commonwealth Avenue.

NITROUS OXID ANALGESIA IN OBSTETRICS

ITS ADVANTAGES OVER THE FREIBURG METHOD

CARL H. DAVIS, M.D.

Assistant Attending Obstetrician and Gynecologist to the Presbyterian
Hospital

CHICAGO

If the belief that pain is an inevitable accompaniment of labor has, in the past, reconciled mothers to endure it, the joy of successful motherhood has caused them to forget it. Severe pain is not essential to childbirth, and there is no logical reason why women should endure it. For many centuries drugs have been used to relieve pain in surgical cases, but it was only sixty-eight years ago that Simpson introduced anesthetics into obstetric practice. Six years later, when Queen Victoria gave them her seal of approval chloroform *a la reine* became the fashion and analgesia was maintained for many hours in large numbers of cases.

DEVELOPMENT OF ANESTHETICS

The development of anesthetics is an interesting chapter in the history of medicine. Sir Humphrey Davy, in 1800, discovered the anesthetic properties of nitrous oxid, and suggested its employment in surgery in the following words: "As nitrous oxid, in its extensive operation, seems capable of destroying physical pain, it may probably be used to advantage during surgical operations in which no great effusion of blood takes place." In 1818, Faraday showed that the inhalation of ether vapor produced anesthetic effects similar to those of nitrous oxid. Crawford W. Long of Georgia, in 1842, used ether to produce anesthesia during surgical operations. Two years later, Horace Wells had a tooth extracted while under the influence of nitrous oxid. Morton used ether for surgical anesthesia in the Massachusetts General Hospital in 1846, and made the first public announcement of its use for this purpose. In January, 1847, Simpson first used ether to produce analgesia in midwifery. Flourens, in March of the same year, announced the anesthetic properties of chloroform, and Simpson, in November, read his paper entitled, "Notice of a New Anesthetic Agent as a Substitute for Sulphuric Ether in Surgery and Midwifery." From this time there was a rapid development of chloroform anesthesia, while after the death of Wells little use was made of nitrous oxid until after Edmund Andrews, in 1863, suggested its use with oxygen.

SCOPOLAMIN AND MORPHIN IN OBSTETRICS

Steinbüchel of Gratz first used scopolamin and morphin for obstetric analgesia in 1903. Gauss published his first results in 1906. The method was tried by many physicians with varying degrees of success, but until the recent visit of Gauss to America and the magazine publicity given his "Dämmerschlaf," the use of scopolamin and morphin did not become a question of vital importance. The magazines have proclaimed to the women of America that no longer shall it be said: "In sorrow thou shall bring forth children." The "Freiburg method" has been used with some degree of success in a large number of cases, but those who have had the largest experience are agreed that this method should be employed only in a well-equipped hospital with a delivery room protected from all noise and confusion. The physician must have had a large experience with the drugs used. The scopolamin must be of a stable brand and freshly prepared. The cases must be carefully selected. Notwithstanding all these precautions, failures are reported in from 10 to 40 per cent. of the cases. From a careful study of the published reports, we are convinced that the "Dämmer-schlaf" is not the panacea the lay press has led our patients to believe. Although this method can never come into general use, the suffering during labor is but the tide in the ocean of motherhood, and the desire of mothers is not for amnesia, but for eutocia.

NITROUS OXID IN OBSTETRICS

Klikowitsch of Petrograd applied nitrous oxid and oxygen analgesia to twenty-five obstetric cases in 1880. He used 80 per cent. nitrous oxid and 20 per cent. oxygen, and observed that three or four inhalations rendered the uterine contractions painless without clouding the consciousness. He reported that the uterine contractions were often stimulated and that in no case was there any diminution in their frequency or strength. Tittel and Doederlein condemned the use of nitrous oxid, but they gave it to the stage of anesthesia and it often caused asphyxia.

J. Clarence Webster was one of the first in America to use nitrous oxid and oxygen in obstetric practice. About ten years ago he began to use it in operative obstetrics when ether and chloroform were contraindicated, and gradually extended its use to all types of cases. In 1909 I gave the anesthetic for him in the first cesarean section which was performed under nitrous oxid and oxygen. During that year we gave this anesthetic for all types of operative obstetrics, and in one primipara gave a few inhalations during each uterine contraction for about two hours prior to a forceps delivery in a case of persistent occipitoposterior position. Although at that time we appreciated the value of nitrous oxid in obstetric practice, its use was largely limited to the end of the second stage, as the hospital was not willing to bear the expense of its prolonged administration. Arthur Guedel, in 1911, advocated the use of nitrous oxid and air analgesia during the second stage of labor; but our first knowledge of its prolonged use in America was in July, 1913, when Drs. Lynch and Hoag attended in confinement the daughter of a Mr. Clark, the maker of a gas-mixing apparatus. In that case, Mr. Clark's demonstrator gave the analgesia for more than six hours. Dr. Lynch was very enthusiastic over the results obtained and since then has used it in nearly all his cases. Dr. Heaney, who began its extended use about the same time, is equally enthusiastic.

It is our custom at the Presbyterian Hospital to begin the analgesia whenever the uterine contractions become painful. If started early in labor, we use a higher percentage of oxygen and give three or four inhalations. Later we use less oxygen and allow five or six deep inhalations previous to the bearing-down effort. The gas must be inhaled with the first suggestion of a contraction; after the patient has made strong traction on the straps, which we fasten to the foot of the bed, she is often given another inhalation containing a larger percentage of oxygen. In giving the analgesia the gas-bags should be only about half filled. The mixture required varies considerably and must be determined for each patient.

To understand nitrous oxid analgesia, you must experiment on yourself. Take six deep inhalations of nitrous oxid and note the effect. Try nitrous oxid and air; and nitrous oxid with various percentages of oxygen; take an inhalation of pure oxygen after securing analgesia. With the knowledge thus obtained you may soon become proficient in its use.

CHOICE OF GAS MACHINE FOR ANALGESIA

A satisfactory analgesia in most cases can be obtained with nitrous oxid and air as has been advocated by Guedel. We have used this method with very good results; but it must be remembered that in giving 20 per cent. air we are supplying 16 per cent. nitrogen, displacing an equal amount of nitrous oxid and delaying the analgesia by at least one inhalation.

For the nitrous-oxid-air analgesia we have a machine with an automatic regulator and a foot control. This apparatus has an advantage over that used by Guedel in that we can maintain a constant pressure in the gas-bag and may control the administration throughout labor without assistance. But after considerable experience with both methods, we are convinced that the better results will be obtained when oxygen is used; and while it necessitates a more expensive apparatus and slightly increases the cost of administering the analgesia, we advise its use. In the maternity ward of the Presbyterian Hospital we are using a mixing apparatus equipped with automatic regulators which enable us to maintain a constant pressure in the gas-bag. These lessen the amount of nitrous oxid and oxygen used. For use in the home I have a similar machine, but on a smaller stand, so that it may be carried easily in an automobile. The mixture of the gases is accomplished with a single dial, so that the nurse or intern, if at the hospital, or some member of the family, if in the home, may readily give the proper mixture. Since we wish the patient to make traction during her pains, self administration is not practical during the latter part of labor, although it may be used in the early part.

COST OF NITROUS OXID-OXYGEN ANALGESIA

By using nitrous oxid and air we have maintained analgesia for three and one-half hours with a 100 gallon tank of gas. After considerable experimenting we have made a hospital charge of $1.50 per hour for the nitrous oxid and oxygen used in maintaining analgesia. As we use the large cylinders, it allows for any leakage and usually gives the hospital a small profit.

In no case has it been necessary to maintain the analgesia for longer than six hours. In multiparas it is rarely necessary to give it for more than two hours. In primiparas the labor is usually terminated in less than three hours from the beginning of the painful

contractions. Should an operative delivery be necessary, the analgesia is increased to anesthesia. Much
depends on the prenatal care of the mother and the
position of the child. In maintaining analgesia the
confidence of the patient is necessary, and mental suggestion is of great value.

ADVANTAGES OF NITROUS OXID–OXYGEN ANALGESIA

Nitrous oxid and oxygen is known to be the safest
of anesthetics. Given to the stage of analgesia it may
be administered with safety over long periods of time.
Nitrous oxid can only cause death by asphyxia. Den-
tists give it to the stage of analgesia to thousands of
patients every year. It is quickly eliminated and has
no deleterious effects on mother or child. In no case
will the analgesia lengthen labor, but rather will
shorten it because of better assistance on the part of
the mother. We concede that it is easier to carry a
hypodermic needle than a gas machine; but the "Freiburg method" may be used only by the specialist, while
nitrous oxid and oxygen analgesia may be employed
safely and efficiently by all who will. It is as safe in
the home as in the hospital. It may be used in all
classes of cases, the results varying with the cooperation of the patient and the skill of the obstetrician. It
gives an increased control over the patient, in that there
are none of the hysterical outbursts so often seen in
the delivery room.

Thirty years ago in speaking of the expectant
mothers, Lusk warned us that: "As the nervous
organization loses in the power of resistance as the
result of higher civilization and of artificial refinement,
it becomes imperatively necessary for the physician to
guard her from the dangers of excessive and too prolonged suffering."

Recent investigations have shown that both chloroform and ether are a source of danger and their use
has been limited to the end of the second stage. In
an alternating series of cases at a Brooklyn hospital,

Allen has shown that the women under scopolamin and morphin are in labor longer and do not feel as well afterward as the women who have the nitrous oxid and oxygen analgesia. Drugs act differently; people have their idiosyncrasies; the hypodermic injection of scopolamin and morphin is beyond recall. But with the nitrous oxid and oxygen analgesia we have eutocia without danger to mother or child. In the use of nitrous oxid and oxygen we have a method which may be used in the home and in the hospital; a method which does not interfere with an aseptic technic.

25 East Washington Street.

MORPHIN AND SCOPOLAMIN AMNESIA IN OBSTETRICS

JOHN OSBORN POLAK, M.D.

Fellow of the American College of Surgeons; Professor of Obstetrics
and Gynecology, Long Island College Hospital

BROOKLYN

Just a year ago, through the publication of an article in the lay press describing painless labor as conducted at Freiburg, the interest of the women of this country was awakened in the so-called "twilight sleep," and since that time women have been calling for its general adoption, while the profession, as a whole, has refused its endorsement, claiming that the merits of the method are not proved. It is my purpose in this brief paper to present the facts, without prejudice or bias, based on a most careful study of this form of amnesia in both Europe and America.

Before taking up a consideration of the method, its indications, advantages, and limitations, we must settle whether a woman is entitled to relief from pain in labor, for some claim that because labor is a physiologic process there is no need of using anything to ameliorate suffering. With this I cannot agree, for physiologic acts are better and more easily performed when one is insensible to physical pain.

"Dämmerschlaf" is a partial narcosis produced by morphin and scopolamin, which should be so light as to eliminate memory of subjective pain without interfering with the uterine contractions. In reality it is an amnesic state in which the patient forgets the successive events in her labor. This effect is produced by individualizing the patient and inducing the "twilight" state, as it is called, by administering an initial dose of $\frac{1}{8}$ or $\frac{1}{4}$ grain of morphin muriate and $\frac{1}{130}$ grain of scopolamin hydrobromid. The morphin is seldom if ever repeated; the scopolamin is repeated in doses of $\frac{1}{400}$ to $\frac{1}{200}$ grain, at varying intervals, until the desired effect is attained. Going into the twilight state is very similar to going under an anesthetic: the personality of the operator, the confidence of the patient, the quiet of the environment, have much to do with the ease of the patient's transition from consciousness to unconsciousness.

The critics of this method claim that it is dangerous to both mother and child; that it does not benefit the patient, for the successes are so few and the effects of the drug so unreliable, that its further trial is not justified; that it prolongs labor; that it provokes post-partum hemorrhage; that it is impossible to maintain an aseptic technic because of the necessity of more frequent examinations to watch the progress of the labor. Also that owing to the delirium and restlessness produced by the drugs it is difficult to maintain the aseptic drapings *in place,* and that the eye and mental symptoms persist in a certain proportion of the cases. All of these criticisms must be refuted or admitted before morphin-scopolamin amnesia can take a place in rational obstetrics.

Dr. Ralph M. Beach and I have studied over four hundred labors under scopolamin-morphin amnesia occurring in our services at Long Island College Hospital, Methodist Episcopal Hospital, and Jewish Hospital, Brooklyn. In this series there has been no maternal mortality, and less than the usual morbidity. No child has been born dead. There has been no case of postpartum hemorrhage following any of these deliveries. A moderate degree of oligopnea has been present in 15 per cent. of the cases. Real asphyxia was noted less frequently than after ordinary labor. Three children died within the first ten days after delivery. All three were necropsied and the following were the pathologic diagnoses:

diaphragmatic hernia with transposition of the viscera; hemorrhage into both suprarenal capsules; and micro-cephalus. The lungs were specially examined for atalectasis, with negative findings. Certainly the most skeptical cannot say that the scopolamin caused these deaths. The condition of the baby at birth and the spontaneity of its first cry are determined by the skill of the operator in producing the "twilight state" with the minimum dosage, and the length of time of the second stage. As Dr. Beach has so admi-rably said: "A certain number of women are destined to need a forceps delivery, twilight or no twilight, and it is poor judgment to wait indefinitely for a spontaneous labor in these cases, to the detriment of the baby."

Our critics say that these are selected cases, which is true. For of all the women who have elected to come to us to deliver them, over 50 per cent. were private patients, either primaparas who feared con-finement under the usual methods, or women who had had previous children with forceps or had had dead-born children after difficult labor, and were willing to make the sacrifice to come to Brooklyn.

These records include eleven cases of cardiovascular disease, in which there had been or was present a break in the cardiac compensation; two cases of exophthalmic goiter; six cases of pulmonary tuber-culosis; eight eclamptics and twenty-two borderline contractions in which a test of labor was given. Hence it will be seen that we have not confined our energies to the normal case and excluded the patho-logic.

To use morphin-scopolamin amnesia properly, cer-tain requisites are necessary: first, a fundamental knowledge of the principles of obstetrics; second, a rational conception of the degree of amnesia to be obtained; third, the attendance of trained operators; fourth, the willingness on the part of the operator to give the time necessary to the proper conduct of the case; and finally, a proper hospital environment. From our experience we cannot comprehend the failures recorded by even good men with this method, unless those in charge of the services do too little and expect too much to secure success. The same sane obstetric principles apply just as much to the conduct of a labor under morphin-scopolamin as when no medicinal aid is used. A woman must have labor pains; the cervix must be dilated; and the presenting part and fetus must be able to pass through the pelvis at both the inlet and outlet, in order that the child may be born. Dilatation takes time and pain, and hundreds of our present-day women tire before this dilatation is complete and are subjected to the trauma consequent on untimely surgical intervention.

We may expect amnesia (no memory of the progress of the labor) in from 70 to 80 per cent. of the cases, and though the patient may have islands of memory, the course of the first stage is always eased and the first stage in primaparas actually shortened. Dilatation of the cervix is promptly effected. This is especially noticeable when the membranes have ruptured early. The greatest advantage gained by the use of scopolamin-morphin is that it affords time for the natural processes to obtain the complete dilatation of the cervix, which admits, if there is any disproportion between the head and the pelvis, that the presenting part is driven farther into the pelvis, and consequently should operative procedures be necessary they are of trivial moment. This to my mind has been conclusively shown by the fact that there has been a great reduction in the median forceps operations, not only in our own clinics but in other clinics in this country in which twilight sleep has been used.

Granting, for the sake of argument, that "dämmerschlaf" is a rational obstetric procedure, what are its indications? It may be used in any labor in which the pains are actually established and there is no marked disproportion between the head and the pelvis. It is especially suitable in long, painful, first-stage labors, or in minor degrees of contraction when it is desirable to give the woman a full test of labor, and in the neurotic women of the mentally and physically unfit class. It is contraindicated in primary uterine inertia, marked pelvic contractions, accidental hemorrhage, placenta praevia, the presence of a dead or dying fetus, as well as in obstetric emergencies, as prolapsed cord, prolapsed arm, and transverse presentations in which the membranes have long been ruptured.

From our experience we can state with reasonable positiveness that this method has certain definite advantages; namely, first, the patient, in from 70 to 80 per cent. of the cases, has a practically painless labor; second, that the nerve exhaustion which comes after prolonged labor is absent when morphin and scopolamin have been used properly; third, that the milk secretion is definitely increased, as shown by the gain in weight of the children in our series; fourth, that the cervix dilates more easily under this form of medication, hence cervical injuries are less frequent; fifth, that the number of midplane forceps operations is diminished; sixth, that the cardiac patients, even when there is some break in compensation, go through labor with a minimum of nervous apprehension and less muscular effort; seventh, the toxemic cases, even with increased blood pressure, go through labor with less likelihood of convulsions, and the urinary output is not affected; and, finally, more babies are born alive owing to the more accurate observation of the fetal heart, and the observance of obstetric indications than is common under ordinary methods. The dangers to the mother are practically nil, to the child the danger is from the prolongation of the second stage due to overdosage, and there is an interrelation between these two.

We have found little difficulty in watching the course of labor by abdominal and rectal examination, and in this way the number of vaginal examinations has been minimized. During the second stage the fetal heart should be auscultated every fifteen minutes and any change in its rhythm or rate noted. A prolonged second stage is injurious to the child and we meet this condition by the application of a tight abdominal binder, forced flexion of the thighs on the abdomen, expressio foetus, pituitary extract when the head is on the pelvic floor, and a median perineotomy in the presence of a rigid perineum. A proper appreciation of these suggestions will minimize even the number of low forceps required to terminate the second stage. The very severe pain of this stage may be relieved by nitrous oxid and oxygen, as suggested by Webster and Lynch, or the employment of a few drops of chloroform.

In the better class of patients there is little or no delirium. In the lower and more ignorant class considerable restlessness is always noted in the second stage. From my personal experience and from the admirable statistics based on 1,000 cases collected by Dr. Beach, which include the work of twenty-six different operators, we can draw the following conclusions:

1. The twilight sleep state is a reality and is applicable in any labor in which there is no primary inertia, marked pelvic contraction, or the presence of obstetric accidents.

2. It is especially applicable to nervous women of the physically unfit type.

3. It is a valuable adjunct in the management of borderline contractions, for it allows the woman a full test of labor.

4. It is distinctly a first-stage procedure and bears the same relation to the first stage as chloroform and nitrous oxid bear to the second stage: it relieves the pain but does not inhibit the progress of labor.

5. It is particularly useful in cardiac cases as it relieves the nervous apprehension and secures dilatation with less muscular effort.

6. It diminishes the shock of labor, whether that labor be normal, prolonged or operative.

7. It does not diminish the milk supply.

8. It does not predispose to postpartum hemorrhage.

9. It does decrease the number of high forceps operations.

And, finally, it has a distinct place in hospital obstetrics, and should be tried out by those who have control of sufficient material definitely to determine its position in obstetric practice.

287 Clinton Avenue.

ABSTRACT OF DISCUSSION
ON PAPERS OF DRS. DAVIS AND POLAK

Dr. WALTER E. LIBBY, Los Angeles: As my experience has been limited to the use of scopolamin and narcophin during labor, my discussion will cover that phase of the subject. This experience is based on forty-two cases observed at the University of California Hospital. Of these cases, twenty-one were multiparas and twenty-one were primiparas. They all had normal pelves and in every case the fetus presented by the vertex. The technic followed was that advocated by Siegel—a definite amount of the drugs at a stated interval. We found that if this schedule was followed implicitly, in some instances the anesthesia was too deep, resulting in asphyxiation of the child. In other words, this method represented the maximum dosage. Believing that the asphyxiation was due to too much narcophin, we have eliminated it except in the first dose. Moreover, we have attempted to individualize each case as to dosage. This has yielded good results and in our last twelve cases not a single case of asphyxia has been encountered. Supplementary anesthesia by chloroform was used, as is our custom, except in eight cases. These exceptions were made in order to demonstrate the effectiveness of the anesthesia. Although none of these patients remembered anything about the delivery, we believe better technic results if chloroform is given. Results of this series are as follows: total number of cases, 42; successful cases, 35, 85 per cent.; partial success, 2, 4 per cent.; failures, 5, 11 per cent.; largest number of doses, 12, covering a period of nineteen hours; average dosage, 5. The effect on the mother was negligible. Excitement which required attention occurred three times. Thirst was observed in about two thirds of the cases, but was never distressing. Muscular twitchings were noted twenty-eight times. Slight acceleration of the pulse rate and other circulatory disturbances of a minor character, such as flushing of the face, were noted. The effect on labor was as follows: 1. Prolongation, multiparas one hour, primiparas two to three hours. The third stage of labor was normal. 2. Pituitary extract was used eleven times, but only four times successfully. In the remaining seven cases forceps were necessary. 3. Forceps were used seven times, 14 per cent.: two times a midforceps and five times a low. The effect on the child varied according to the dosage. Alarming asphyxia occurred six times and all of these patients required resuscitation with hot and cold water for a period of fifteen to thirty minutes. Since our change in technic deep asphyxia has been absent. One fetal death occurred and necropsy revealed a perforate intraventricular septum, stenosis of the pulmonary valve with dilatation of the pulmonary artery and hypertrophy and dilatation of the heart. No detrimental effect on the child during the puerperium was noted.

Dr. W. Francis B. Wakefield, San Francisco: I have confined my eighty-one patients under scopolamin anesthesia. I am sorry because Dr. Davis chose exactly the title that he did for his paper. I think it is to be deprecated that we should make comparisons that might, perhaps, have an influence on the minds of those listening to us, between one good method and another good method. It is evident to me that Dr. Davis has had no personal experience with scopolamin as an anesthetic in labor, and that he has had a great deal of useful experience with nitrous oxid. The same thing may perhaps hold true with Dr. Polak, with the thing reversed. I think it is high time that the American obstetricians were willing to try out these different methods of ameliorating the pain of childbirth and let each one choose the one which appeals most strongly to him, and which has given the best results in his individual experience. So far as I am concerned, I have been using for the last thirteen months, in my private work entirely, scopolamin amnesia, and it has given me thoroughly satisfactory results. I can concur in almost every statement that Dr. Polak has made. I don't see why he excludes the women with dead babies from participating in these benefits. I have had two women who came to me within the last month, in both of whom there was every evidence of a dead fetus, and the history in the first case would show that the fetus had been dead ten days, and in the second case eight. In these I induced labor and put them under scopolamin anesthesia as in the others, because I see no reason why they should be deprived of painless labor. I cannot agree with Dr. Davis when he says that the statements that have been made in the public press for the most part are erroneous. I believe that the *Dämmerschlaf*, properly used, does carry out practically all the rational statements made in the popular press.

When I speak of the "twilight sleep" I wish to speak of one single technic which originated at Freiburg, the Gauss technic, and no other. There has been a lot of work done in a haphazard kind of way with other forms of technic, using scopolamin as a basis, and some of the results have been very bad. I cannot agree with the statement of Dr. Davis that these patients, after scopolamin amnesia, did not feel as well as with nitrous oxid. I have used nitrous oxid to some extent, and one of the most remarkable things about the scopolamin amnesia is that these patients, when they waken from the sleep (and it is a couple of hours before they wake up; we let them have their sleep out), wake with all their vital forces thoroughly aroused. They feel good and strong and active and I have great difficulty in keeping most of these women in bed twenty-four hours.

DR. JENNINGS CRAWFORD LITZENBURG, Minneapolis: I think perhaps, I am in an enviable position. None of the gentlemen who have spoken here have had experience with both methods; I have. After I returned from Europe I thought it the duty of every man with a clinic to experiment with the *Dämmerschlaf*. This has been done for the past several months in the University Hospital in Minneapolis.

Some difficulty has been experienced in keeping my associate from becoming overenthusiastic. We have to warn ourselves continually that our series is small; it is yet less than one hundred. However, I cannot quite understand some of the dire results that have been obtained in some other hospitals, or why certain hospitals in this country have forbidden the use of the *Dämmerschlaf*, because our results have been, as far as we have gone, satisfactory. The series is so small that we are not willing to draw final conclusions. I am simply reporting the results. They are about the same as Dr. Polak's: about 15 per cent. of failures or practical failures and no fatally asphyxiated children. Only three had to be tubbed for asphyxiation; sometimes there was only very mild delirium in the mother.

In the use of nitrous oxid my experience has been delightful. The women are enthusiastic about it. They also have the "twilight" condition. The next day, even though they had complained during the labor, they say they have forgotten that they did and that they knew they were bearing down, but that they felt no pain whatever. In other words, there is a twilight condition with the nitrous oxid. I have been averse to using it in the private home, because in all my work I have had the expert anesthetists of the hospital give it, and only in the hospital, and I would like to ask Dr. Davis if his statements about the small danger of it can reasonably be true. I have felt with the experience we have had in surgery perhaps there might be some danger with the nitrous oxid in unskilled hands. Allow me to say that it shortens labor. Recently while in Chicago, I had the pleasure of investigating the work being done by Dr. Davis, Dr. Lynch and Dr. Heaney. While I was away a woman who had a right occipitoposterior presentation was in labor the two days I was gone under care of an expert obstetrician who called me on my return. I gave nitrous oxid. With her second pain after taking the nitrous oxid she began to bear down hard, and in four and a half hours she was delivered spontaneously, with the complete rotation of the head. Nitrous oxid has the additional advantage of 100 per cent. success. You relieve the pain of all of them. There is not that 15 per cent. of failure. I have used a combination of the two methods—*dämmerschlaf* during the first stage, giving only two doses of scopolamin, gr. 1/144, and one dose of morphin, ⅙ or ⅛, and thereafter nitrous oxid whenever the woman begins to complain, continuing throughout the labor. I commend this procedure for trial.

DR. CARL G. PARSONS, Denver: As a professional anesthetist for the last twelve years, I have had a good deal of experience in all sorts of anesthesia and also in *Dämmerschlaf* (Gauss method).

The various ways of administration and dosages of scopolamin have tended to bewilder the profession, so it seems pertinent to outline the different methods of use of this drug alone or in conjunction with other drugs: 1. As a preliminary to anesthesia, both local and general. 2. As a true hypodermic anesthetic (surgical anesthesia) without the addition of any inhalation anesthetic. 3. As *Dämmerschlaf* (Krönig-Gauss-Freiburg method). 4. Innumerable modifications of No. 3. 5. When given for therapeutic purposes.

DR. CARL L. HOAG, San Francisco: Dr. Davis in his admirable paper has not given us any information as to the degree of relaxation of the perineal muscles under nitrous oxid and oxygen compared with that obtained when using chloroform or ether. From my rather extensive experience with nitrous oxid and oxygen in the surgical field, I should say that the main reason why this anesthetic has not rapidly supplanted the others is that by itself it does not give sufficient muscular relaxation. A similar failure of relaxation in the perineal muscles would greatly increase the risk of tearing and might offset any other advantages the new anesthesia might have over the old. The added feature that makes nitrous oxid and oxygen the anesthetic of choice in surgery is the local blocking of impulses from the operative area to the brain—

Crile's "anociassociation." In the early part of this year I began to apply this principle in the obstetric field. Using nitrous oxid and oxygen as Dr. Davis has described; when the head begins to distend the perineum in the second stage, the vulval edges are turned back and the levator ani muscles and perineal body are thoroughly injected with novocain. When this is well done the effect is striking. The same relaxation can be secured here as in the abdominal muscles. The injection of this region with novocain has been done so many times in rectal and perineal operations that we need not fear edema, hematoma, infections or delayed healing. The effects of the drug on the child must be slight, if any. Similar amounts have been used without deleterious effects in many cesarean sections.

Dr. L. I. Breitstein, San Francisco: These methods of anesthesia are very important and have merit. They should be used when properly indicated. No one should limit himself to a routine method. Each case should be individualized and the form of anesthesia best suited to the case in hand should be employed. For instance, in dealing with a primipara—one who is full of fear, who cannot stand pain, who is of an hysterical nature—morphin-scopolamin anesthesia is best suited in that particular case, because these drugs have a selective action when it comes to allay fear and produce amnesia. On the other hand, in a multipara who has had three or four children, whose soft parts are relaxed and who has short labors, the anesthetic of choice would be a few whiffs of chloroform as the head passes over the perineum. It is ridiculous to try to give such women the "twilight sleep." Furthermore, take the cases you see for the first time at the end of the first stage of labor, or during the second stage; these cases are best treated with the nitrous oxid and oxygen method. You have to individualize your cases. My experience with nitrous oxid and oxygen has been limited to seven cases and my only objection has been the expense. Dr. Davis spoke of the ridiculously low cost for the administration of nitrous oxid and oxygen. My experience has been otherwise.

The prospective mother now consults the obstetrician early to find out if her particular case is suitable for the "twilight sleep." She has been informed that certain examinations —urine, blood pressure, etc.—are necessary. She knows that these examinations have to be made at regular intervals. In other words, we get the patients early and we can give them good prenatal care. During labor the condition of the fetus is ascertained by repeated examinations. The constant presence of the obstetrician insures early detection of complications. I do not wish to be misunderstood; I make it understood that obstetric anesthesia is not a panacea for all obstetric complications that are apt to arise.

Dr. M. W. Kapp, San Jose, Calif.: I am one of the little fellows from the country, without a hospital or the material to give the nitrous oxid. I have not the help always to give the *Dämmerschlaf* treatment, but I have had experience with another line with which I have had broad success. I have found something that for four years I have used with perfect success and safety. It is so ridiculously simple that you will laugh at it, but try it some time when you are all alone and the woman crying out in agony. It is heroin, and it will work in every case except in uterine inertia. I have used it in about 140 cases. Heroin one-twelfth grain hypodermically as soon as the pains become severe, no matter what stage of labor. You get the full effect in fifteen or twenty minutes and it will relieve the patient be she primipara or multipara. It does not produce amnesia but it does produce sufficient analgesic effect so that the patient will "rise up and call you blessed."

Dr. E. M. Lazard, Los Angeles: On hearing the favorable reports of those who have preceded me, I wonder why the *Dämmerschlaf* has not been adopted by all the practitioners throughout the country. I am the more diffident in speaking on this subject after a remark by one of the preceding speakers that usually a critic does not know what he is talking about. I have had no experience with the *Dämmerschlaf*; frankly, I have been afraid of it; I felt that the claims of the lay journals were, to say the least, overdone. Some of the points of doubt in my mind have not been changed by the speakers this afternoon, and I would like to ask a question or two. The impression prevails among the laity that all women should have the benefit of the *Dämmerschlaf*. In Harrar and MacPherson's report they say that to not more than 25 per cent. of the women that come into the hospital in labor can they apply this, because the labor is too far advanced, and in that 25 per cent. of cases they have only 70 per cent. success. I would like to ask Dr. Polak to what percentage of women who come into his lying-in clinics in labor is the method applicable? Nothing has been said as to the memory test. Krönig and Gauss lay particular stress on this portion of the technic, saying that the entire method must stand or fall by the memory test. If I am not mistaken, Dr. Wakefield, who has spoken, and who has reported favorably on his cases, has done away entirely with the memory test. Am I correct, Dr. Wakefield?

Dr. Wakefield: That is correct.

Dr. Lazard: I would not call that the Freiburg technic, because the Freiburg authorities insist on the memory test as a control of dosage; so nearly every observer has some modification of the method as elaborated at Freiburg. From reports from the various clinics we hear of wild delirium, and this question has been minimized by the speakers. I would like to ask them what their experience in this regard has been. The Michael Reese Hospital gave the method a thorough trial, and, in THE JOURNAL, gave, as you probably all know, a very unfavorable report of their experience. Dr. Frankenthal, who is in charge there, had made the suggestion that possibly an impending rupture of the uterus might be covered up by the drugs, and in their series they report one case with rupture of the uterus with a fatal ending. This was not considered due to the drug, but there would appear to be less likelihood of detecting symptoms of an impending rupture with a patient under *Dämmerschlaf*.

DR. L. M. GATES, Scranton, Pa.: Like all new methods, there has been a constantly changing technic, and it is the early technic with the large and repeated doses of morphin that caused the death of the babies. If that is the case, cannot we, by some other method produce the same results? I would suggest first the use of scopolamin; then, if you need morphin, use it later. I have tried it and find you can accomplish the results without the use of morphin. In one case recently, that of a weak patient with a poor heart and valvular lesion, a decided blonde to whom I did not desire to give morphin, crying for help, I gave 1/200 grain of scopolamin. She quieted down and worked hard and it accomplished the same result. If heroin is better than morphin, why not use it, and in small doses along with scopolamin?

DR. HUGH S. MOUNT, Oregon City, Ore.: I concur in the remarks of Dr. Polak on "twilight sleep." I do not wish to go into details of cases, but we have had excellent results.

If the general practitioner feels that he can use "twilight sleep" and make a success of it, he is mistaken. He will have to give up his other practice, because he will have to sit on the job from the time labor starts until it is finished; that has been our experience. It ties you up for fifteen to twenty hours, and you have to know every minute what the mother is doing, and the baby as well. You have to have a history of every pain. Who is there in general or surgical practice that wants to take a case like this and sit down to make the history? It is a fine thing for the mothers, and if it does nothing else, will raise the standard of obstetrics.

This country is being flooded with proprietary drug preparations, to which the President of the Association called our attention this morning. There have been several representatives of this class to see me who have "twilight sleep" put up in tablets, principally morphin, and they say they make *real* "twilight sleep." I want to call your attention to the fact that these are dangerous, and I have no more respect for the physician that would give repeated doses of these than for the one who would give a pound bottle of chloroform to the husband with instructions to use it when labor begins.

"Twilight sleep" is a good thing in the hands of those who have the time and technic for it. Every woman who takes it wants it again; even if amnesia be not complete, they desire the relief from the mental suffering that it gives.

DR. WM. R. LIVINGSTON, Oxnard, Calif.: I have had about forty-five cases in which I employed "twilight sleep" since my return from Freiburg last autumn, and the results have been very satisfactory. A constant surprise to us has been the condition of these women postpartum. Following these labors there seems to be an entire absence of the customary shock. To further this, we are careful that the post delivery sleep is as long as possible. On the following day there is difficulty in keeping these patients in bed, and we usually get them up on the second or third day. In every consideration of the subject of "twilight sleep" we should recognize, first, that there is a technic of Gauss, with individualization of the patient, and in which the dose of morphin or other opium derivative is seldom repeated; second, that there is a technic of Siegel, with a prearranged schedule, and that this was an experimental attempt to standardize the treatment; third, the use of morphin with each injection of scopolamin is sometimes wrongly spoken of as "twilight sleep"; and fourth, there is a tendency to use the term "twilight sleep" in any treatment in which some opium derivative, as for instance, heroin, is given alone. These different procedures must not be confused if we are to have any definite understanding of the subject. I believe most of the men who have had favorable results have followed the method of Gauss. I think those who have followed Siegel's technic have found it unsatisfactory, because they did not individualize the patients. The attempt to follow this prearranged schedule is the probable reason for the unsatisfactory reports of some of the earlier cases. I believe we are all coming to the individualization method of Gauss.

DR. CARL H. DAVIS, Chicago: I have no intention of condemning the use of scopolamin and morphin when it is used at the patient's request, and according to the method outlined by Gauss. If we are to believe the public results of Gauss and other observers, its use by the general practitioner must be condemned. It would be splendid if every woman could go into an especially equipped hospital for confinement. We hope that the obstetric standards will greatly improve, and that large endowments may be secured for maternity hospitals. But at present few women are delivered by the obstetric specialist, and a method which cannot be used safely by the general practitioner will be of no assistance to most mothers.

Nitrous oxid and oxygen analgesia has in our hands relieved the suffering in every case. Since we only give from four to six deep inhalations in securing analgesia, the assistance of a trained anesthetist is not necessary, provided one uses a simple apparatus such as we use at the Presbyterian Hospital. As stated in the paper, we can maintain analgesia for more than three hours with a hundred gallon tank of nitrous oxid. While the cost is increased by using the small tanks which must be employed in the homes, the cost should average from four to six dollars and rarely exceed twelve dollars. But you must be careful not to allow a leakage, as it will prove expensive. I find that most patients are willing to pay for the gas.

A combination of two methods, as was suggested by Drs. Polak and Litzenburg, may be of value in selected cases. The use of morphin or heroin either alone or combined with chloral hydrate has long been employed in cases with a protracted first stage. It is possible that the scopolamin might be better than the chloral. We have not had occasion to combine the methods although our staff have discussed its possibilities.

The perineal injection of novocain has been used in Chicago. About a year ago M. L. Harris blocked the nerve and did a low forceps delivery. Dr. Heaney has used it in combination with the nitrous oxid analgesia. While it is of great help in destroying the pain, I fear that it might increase the number of lacerations. The combination of nitrous oxid and oxygen analgesia with the local anesthesia with $\frac{1}{200}$ grain novocain is the ideal anesthetic for cesarean section. I trust that during the next year the members of this section will try the nitrous oxid and oxygen analgesia. In selected cases try the combined methods, but remember that it is rarely necessary.

DR. JOHN O. POLAK, Brooklyn: It seems that those men who are really trying this method are beginning to come to the belief that there is something in it. The unfortunate position that we have been in in the East has been that those who would not try it damned it, and those who tried it lauded it. I agree absolutely with those who said we should individualize each patient. It is only a small proportion of the patients brought into our maternity service by the ambulance on which this method can be used. It is the patients whom we send in at the expected date or a few days before on which we use this method throughout, for the reason that the patient cannot be too far advanced in labor if we are to get a good amnesia. The danger is the prolonged second stage. We have obviated this by not using it or beginning it too close to the beginning of the second stage. We practically discontinue the method and substitute either gas and oxygen or chloroform for the second stage. This continues the amnesia produced by the scopolamin. In other words, we have done what Crile does: given them their preoperative doses of morphin and scopolamin.

The danger to the child is threefold: (1) overdosage; (2) in interference with the uteroplacental circulation after the rupture of the membranes; and (3) the prolongation of the second stage due to the breaking of the rules of obstetric procedure, that is, letting the second stage go beyond two or two and a half hours.

We are holding a necropsy on every baby that dies, and are learning that babies die from causes independent of the anesthetic and nonclosure of the foramen ovale. It is for this reason that I said in my paper that we would not give it in case there was a dead or dying child.

We test the memory by noting whether the patient remembers the last hypodermic injection. If the patient has lost memory of the last hypodermic injection and does not know when that was given or how many injections she has had— we do not try to wake her up by dolls or watches or anything of that sort.

We have had a few cases of delirium just as the head was passing over the perineum. This has been in foreign women. In the better class of women we have had practically no delirium. These patients go to sleep and wake up three hours afterwards, with no bad results.

TUBERCULOSIS OF THE UTERINE APPENDAGES

HOWARD CANNING TAYLOR, M.D.

NEW YORK

CAUSES

General: Tuberculosis of the uterine appendages is usually secondary to a tuberculous infection in another organ. It can be stated, therefore, that anything that predisposes to tuberculosis in general, predisposes to tuberculosis of the genital organs. This may be family disposition, mode of living, race, etc.

Predisposing: Previous gonorrheal infection of the fallopian tubes is claimed to be a predisposing cause of tuberculous salpingitis. In other organs a simple inflammation doubtless predisposes to a tuberculous infection. In the joints, lungs, pleura and elsewhere a simple inflammation frequently precedes a tuberculous infection, and by analogy it can be assumed that the same is true in the appendages. It is unusual to find gonococci in tuberculous appendages, but this does not prove that they may not have been present at the beginning of the process. That gonorrheal infection does not always precede the tuberculous infection is proved by the frequency of the latter in virgins. It is probable that any other inflammation of the appendages, such, for example, as might result from an abortion or childbirth would predispose to a tuberculous infection in the same way.

If it is true that in many cases of tuberculosis of the uterine appendages the infection reaches the tube by direct extension, either from the peritoneum or from the uterine cavity, then a moderate infection would be more frequently followed by a tuberculous process than the more extensive infection leading to occlusion of the uterine and fimbriated ends of the tubes. It is probable even after both ends of the tube have been occluded that the tuberculous infection can occur either through the lymphatic or blood supply, but it is less likely to result from a direct extension. A tuberculous infection on a hydrosalpinx has been reported. Even though the appendages are occluded, the peritoneal coats may be involved by extension in a general peritoneal tuberculosis.

Congenital deformities and malformation of the appendages predispose to tuberculous infection, according to Sellheim, Freund and other authors. In this class would be included cases of infantile uterus. A number of observers have called attention to the frequency with which an abnormally small uterus is found in cases of tuberculosis of the fallopian tubes.

The puerperal uterus is more likely to become infected with tubercle bacilli than the normal uterus. It has been found that the placental site is more frequently infected than other parts of the uterine cavity. From the uterine tuberculosis the appendages may become secondarily infected. In this indirect way, pregnancies would predispose to tuberculous salpingitis.

Ovarian cysts are sometimes found to have a tuberculous infection implanted on the new growth. I have seen one case in which a fibroma of the uterus was involved in a tuberculous process. It is not probable, however, that either ovarian cysts or uterine fibromas should be considered to be predisposing causes of genital tuberculosis.

FREQUENCY

The frequency with which tuberculosis is found in the uterine appendages depends largely on the regularity with which these organs are subjected to a microscopic examination. If the nature of the process is determined only by the gross examination, the number of cases of tubal tuberculosis reported will be small; if, however, every tube and ovary that is removed is examined microscopically, the number will be found to be surprisingly large. It is probable also that the frequency of genital tuberculosis, as tuberculosis of other organs, varies in different locations and among different people. If gonorrheal salpingitis predisposes to tuberculous salpingitis, as it probably does, then naturally tubal tuberculosis will be found more frequently among the class most frequently subject to the former disease.

Krönig, in a series of 400 appendages removed for chronic inflammation, found tuberculosis in 11.5 per cent. of the cases. If in the series, there were also included the cases in which there was a general tuberculous peritonitis with the involvement of the tubes only on the peritoneal coat, there would have been 22 per cent. of tuberculosis. It is probable, as has been suggested, that the actual number is still larger, because in some old healed cases, the tuberculosis might have been overlooked.

Studdiford found tuberculosis in 6 per cent. of tubes removed for inflammatory conditions.

In my own cases tuberculosis was found by routine examination in 5 per cent. of tubes removed for inflammatory conditions. This represented about 2 per cent. of all abdominal operations.

While statistics of different clinics vary, it is probable that at least 10 per cent. of all inflammatory diseases of the uterine appendages are of tuberculous origin.

The ovary is affected by tuberculosis less frequently than the fallopian tube. It is not possible to give the ratio of frequency with which the two organs are affected. Tuberculosis of the ovary cannot always be detected by macroscopic examination, and frequently the ovary, if apparently not diseased, is not removed with the tube.

As the ovary is most frequently involved by extension from the fallopian tube, the stage of the disease at which the cases are examined would modify the ratio of frequency. This would be seen particularly in comparing operative and necropsy cases. In the late necropsy cases, the ovary would be more frequently involved with the tube than in the earlier operative cases. Different observers estimate that the ovary was jointly involved in 10 to 60 per cent. of cases of tuberculosis of the tubes. In my own cases, the ovaries were involved in 22 per cent. of the cases.

Tuberculosis of the ovary without involvement of the tube is exceedingly rare. No such case is reported among my cases.

The extension of the tuberculosis process from the tube to the uterus is of frequent occurrence. Simmons, as reported by Krönig, found the combination of uterine and tubal tuberculosis in 52, or 65 per cent. of 80 necropsies for genital tuberculosis. This does not mean that in all of these cases, the tuberculous process extended from the tube to the uterus. In a certain number, doubtless the tuberculosis existed first in the uterus and later extended to the tube. Kroenig believes that the combination occurs in about one-half of all cases of genital tuberculosis. This fact is an indication for the removal of the uterus if the appendages are removed for tuberculosis.

SOURCES OF INFECTION

There are three modes of infection in genital tuberculosis. They are: (1) through the blood and lymphatic systems; (2) from neighboring organs; (3) by ascending infection through the vagina.

1. Through the blood and lymphatic systems from a tuberculous focus elsewhere, undoubtedly the greatest number of cases occur. The primary focus is most frequently in the lungs, but may be in any of the other organs. The importance of this mode of infection is illustrated by the claim of some observers that no case of undoubted primary tuberculosis of the uterine appendages occurs in the literature.

2. From neighboring organs the uterine appendages are frequently infected by a tuberculosis process. This most frequently occurs from the peritoneum. Frequently the involvement of the peritoneum and the abdominal organs including the uterus and appendages is so general that it is not possible to determine in which place the disease had its origin. That is, whether the tuberculosis started in the appendages and extended from them to the peritoneum, or whether it started in the peritoneum and involved the appendages secondarily. Most observers believe that the peritoneum is the site of the primary lesion.

Kraus reported a case of tuberculosis of the right uterine appendage in which the infection apparently extended from a tuberculous appendix to the fallopian tube. I recently had under my care a persistent sinus following the removal of the appendix. At the operation, I removed a tuberculous pyosalpinx from the bottom of this sinus. I have been unable to learn from the previous operator the exact nature of the original trouble in the appendix.

3. By ascending infection is meant the involvement of the uterus and appendages from infection introduced into the vagina. It has been questioned that tuberculosis of the uterus or of the uterine appendages can result from tubercle bacilli introduced from without into the vagina. In general there are two methods by which tubercle bacilli may be introduced into the vagina — one by coitus with a man with tuberculosis of the testes or seminal tracts, and the other by fingers, soiled instruments, linen, etc., of a person infected with tuberculosis. Against this mode of infection, it has been stated that the tubercle bacilli are destroyed by the vaginal secretions. Also that even if they were deposited in the vagina and remained alive, they could not gain entrance into the uterus and certainly not into the fallopian tubes.

Menge does not accept these views. By mixing vaginal secretions with a solution of tubercle bacilli under conditions resembling those in the vagina, he found that the bacilli were killed. If, however, the solution was diluted, the bacilli remained alive for a number of days. Menge considered this proof that tubercle bacilli in the semen would be protected from the action of the vaginal secretions by dilution. He also believes that the motion of the spermatozoa is sufficient to carry the tubercle bacilli into the uterus and even into the tubes.

Menge also experimentally produced tuberculosis of the uterus in guinea-pigs by injecting a solution containing tubercle bacilli into the seminal vesicles of the male before intercourse.

Bennecke, experimenting on rabbits, was also able to produce tuberculosis of the genital tract by ascending infection.

These experiments of Menge, Bennecke and others would seem to prove that it is possible that infection of the genital tract by tubercle bacilli introduced into the vagina during intercourse is certainly possible. It is, however, doubtful that it is of frequent occurrence. On the other side Blau (quoted by Bennecke) and Sugimura were unable to produce a genital tuberculosis by ascending infection and doubted its occurrence. Krönig believes that an ascending infection from the vagina probably never occurs.

PROGNOSIS

Indication for Operation: Tuberculosis of the uterine appendages is ordinarily a secondary infection. In nearly every case there is elsewhere in the body one or more tuberculous foci; that is, the genital tuberculosis is a part of a more or less general systemic infection.

In order properly to consider the treatment it is necessary to understand the influence which the tuberculous salpingitis exerts in this general process (1) on the life of the patient, (2) on the health of the patient and (3) on the extension of the infection.

The influence of the tuberculous salpingitis on the life of the patient is comparable to that of other forms of salpingitis. Tuberculous salpingitis is rarely the direct cause of death, neither are other forms of salpingitis. In 64 cases of genital tuberculosis found at necropsy in the pathologic laboratory at Freiburg, the genital tuberculosis was not considered the cause of death in any case. This confirms our clinical experience. Very rarely does a tuberculous salpingitis alone seem to be the cause of death. Theoretically we would not expect it to be. The tubes and ovaries are not necessary to life, and their destruction does not in itself materially affect the health of the patient. It is probable, therefore, that it is rarely necessary to operate in a case of tuberculous salpingitis in order to save the life of the patient.

A more difficult problem is to estimate the tendency which the tuberculosis in the appendages has to extend locally or to produce a general systemic infection. There is no doubt that many cases of tuberculous salpingitis subside and are found only at operations for other conditions or at necropsy. That is, that there are healed tuberculous lesions in the tubes and ovaries as in other organs.

The frequency with which a tuberculous salpingitis produces a general peritoneal tuberculosis is still in dispute. Some observers believe that it is the usual rule that the peritoneal infection is from the tube and advocate the removal of the uterus and both appendages for tuberculous salpingitis to prevent the occurrence of tuberculous peritonitis.

The weight of evidence is against this extension. It is probable that a tuberculous inflammation in the tube would cause the formation of adhesions about it in the same way as other types of salpingitis. These adhesions would tend to localize the infection and prevent the general peritoneal tuberculosis. As is known there is a tendency for any minute foreign body in the peritoneal cavity to be carried into the lumen of the tube in the same way that the ova may be. It is possible that the tuberculous infection can be carried in the same way into the tube. Theoretically, therefore, we would expect the tube to be infected from the peritoneum and not the general peritoneal cavity from the tube.

There is ample clinical evidence that an active tuberculous salpingitis does not always infect the peritoneum. Frequently one tube is removed for an inflammatory condition, and the other, diseased to a less extent, is not removed. A microscopic examination proved the excised tube to be tuberculous. It is a fair assumption that the inflammation of the tube that was not removed was of the same nature. In their subsequent course these cases rarely show any signs of a tuberculous peritonitis. Krönig reported twelve consecutive cases of this kind, in none of which apparently did the peritoneum become infected. He believes that the tuberculosis rarely extends from the tube to cause a general peritoneal tuberculosis.

The frequency with which healed tuberculous lesions are found in the tubes with apparently normal peritoneum is additional evidence that tuberculosis of the tubes does not usually extend to the peritoneum.

The frequency of the extension of a tuberculosis of the tubes and ovaries to bladder and intestines is also difficult to determine. Krönig holds that it infrequently extends to these organs and rarely is the starting point of a general miliary tuberculosis. In none of my cases were the intestines or bladder apparently involved. There certainly were no fistulas. Other observers, for example Menge, believe that there is a strong tendency to both local and general extension.

Krönig, believing that tuberculous salpingitis rarely extends, disapproves of operation to prevent such occurrences. Menge, holding the opposite view, operates far more frequently on cases of tuberculous salpingitis.

Practically there is no absolute rule regarding operation for tuberculous salpingitis to prevent a local or general extension. Some cases will remain quiescent or subside, others will progress. If by proper treatment the symptoms subside and the infection is not extending, I prefer to delay operation. If the disease is progressing then an operation is indicated.

The influence of a tuberculous salpingitis on the general health in itself is usually not great. The disease usually runs a chronic course and frequently gives no local or general symptoms. In other cases, it runs a chronic course without local or general symptoms excepting during acute exacerbations. In other cases the symptoms may be constant and possibly severe. In other words, with regard to symptoms, tuberculous salpingitis follows closely a salpingitis from other causes, and has in general the same indications for operation.

The ultimate value of the tube must also be considered in deciding on the treatment of tuberculous salpingitis. It is theoretically possible for a tuberculous salpingitis to subside, leaving a patent tube and allowing the patient to become pregnant. It is doubtful if this often occurs. Furthermore, it is doubtful if it is wise that such a patient should become pregnant for fear of starting again the tuberculous process. There is, therefore, no indication to delay an operation otherwise indicated in order to conserve the tube.

TREATMENT

The treatment of tuberculous peritonitis is not properly included in this paper, and it will be considered only as it is necessary to do so in describing the treatment of tuberculous salpingitis.

The treatment of tuberculous salpingitis will be considered under two classes: (1) those cases in which the tube is involved as a part of the general peritoneal tuberculosis and (2) those cases in which there is only a local peritoneal involvement.

If there is a general peritoneal tuberculosis, that and not the salpingitis is the condition that determines the treatment. If, however, the abdomen is opened for such a condition, usually the tubes, if accessible, should be removed. The chances of the tubes becoming diseased from the peritoneum is so great and the chances of regaining their function so small that they should not be retained. If inaccessible they should not be removed unless they are distended, because the additional peritoneal traumatism necessitated by the removal of the tubes would increase the chances of infection. If the tubes are distended, it is usually best to remove them even if covered by adhesions.

The treatment of the uterus and ovaries depends on their condition and the case. At or approaching the menopause, they should be removed. If the ovaries are diseased they should be removed. If the ovaries are removed the uterus should be also.

If there is no general peritoneal tuberculosis, the treatment of the tuberculous salpingitis is practically the same as for other forms of salpingitis. This is true because if there is no general peritoneal tuberculosis, it is practically impossible to diagnose a tuberculous salpingitis from other varieties.

During the acute stage, or during an acute exacerbation, there should be rest in bed, local applications of ice, proper diet, air, etc. Later there should be local treatment and especial attention to general health. There is no doubt that in this way many cases are completely and permanently cured symptomatically without the diagnosis of tuberculous infection being made or suspected.

After the acute symptoms have subsided, if a distended tube, that is, a tuberculous pyosalpinx remains, or if the acute symptoms are too frequently repeated, then an operation is indicated. The indications for operation are practically the same as for other forms of salpingitis.

At the operation no attempt should be made to save any part of either tube. Usually (90 per cent. of cases) both tubes are involved.

If the ovaries are diseased, or if the patient is near the menopause, the ovaries should be removed.

If the ovaries are removed or if the patient is near the menopause, the uterus should also be removed. It is difficult to decide regarding the uterus in young women with normal ovaries. It has been stated that 50 per cent. of cases of tuberculous salpingitis are associated with tuberculosis of the fundus uteri. There is some risk in not removing this tuberculous focus if it is present. There is also a definite risk of mental and physical discomfort if the ovaries and uterus are removed in young women.

I have not removed the uterus in a number of these cases (often the diagnosis of a tuberculous salpingitis was made only by the microscopic examination) and in no known case has there been subsequent trouble.

The postoperative treatment of tuberculous salpingitis is important. The probability of other tuberculous foci, and the personal predisposition of the patient are indications for the best hygienic surroundings with regard to rest, food, air, etc.

32 West Fiftieth Street.

ABSTRACT OF DISCUSSION

DR. PHILEMON E. TRUESDALE, Fall River, Mass.: The study of any obscure disease is always interesting. Tubal tuberculosis is not only clinically obscure, but its true pathology is occasionally overlooked when the lesion is in plain sight. The affected tubes, particularly in the early stages, have certain characteristics which may be well to mention. In the first place, the original focus is always in the ampulla of the tube. As this develops, the process goes on toward the uterine end of the tube in the production of small nodes, invading the stroma of the tube. There is a more or less characteristic appearance of the fimbriated extremity. The fimbriae are short, thick and have a rosette appearance. Until the tube becomes extensively involved and adherent to surrounding structures, the distal end remains patent and presents often this characteristic appearance.

Dr. Taylor has allowed a very liberal latitude for other views. His observations, however, are based on a large experience and are strengthened by the opinions of the master gynecologist, Krönig. They would, therefore, undeniably, be the truest guides. I have held a belief that tuberculous peritonitis is often the manifestation of a primary focus in the tube. This belief is founded on the experiments of Murphy, the clinical experience of the Mayos, and my own more limited observations. Murphy injected tuberculous material into the free peritoneal cavity of the monkey. This gravitated to the floor of the pelvis and produced a peritonitis. In no case was the stroma of the tubes involved. Dr. Mayo reported seven cases in which the patients had been operated on from one to four times, in which he cleared up the peritonitis by removing the tubes. In a few cases we have found tuberculosis in the tubes and a peritonitis somewhat circumscribed, indicating an extension by continuity. One of these patients I operated on for what appeared to be a chronic appendicitis. At the operation there was a little free fluid, which did not appear to be consistent with the process in the appendix. On further examination the terminal end of the ileum was found studded with small tubercles and both tubes were tuberculous. The tuberculous peritonitis in this case was limited to the peritoneum of the pelvis. However, the value of this discussion rests in the fact that the fallopian tubes should always be examined when the abdomen is opened for tuberculous peritonitis.

In some of the more advanced cases it seems to me well to mention the importance of not doing anything surgically. Dr. Taylor has mentioned the fact that the disease rarely, if ever, is the cause of death, while it is limited to the pelvis. Occasionally, the picture at operation is a fused mass with adhesions extensively involving the intestine. Great danger of fistulae and of miliary tuberculosis here accompanies the removal of the disease. So it seems to me to be the part of wisdom occasionally not to proceed with any surgical interference.

I believe that gauze drains should not be used in these cases, except as a temporary expedient to control hemorrhage. Rubber tissue answers the purpose fully and should be employed when any drain is necessary. When the question of drainage is in doubt, I should be inclined to take the risk against the use of any drain.

Dr. J. E. Engstad, Minneapolis: Dr. Taylor did not mention the bovine and human types of tubercle bacilli. I believe that the tuberculous infection in the peritoneal cavity is due to the bovine type. Both types may exist in the human simultaneously. I believe that in most cases the infection is hematogenous, the primary foci being in the lungs, in the cervical glands or elsewhere. Infection of the uterine appendages is often due to a primary infection of the appendix. In a large number of cases of chronic appendicitis the causative factor is tubercle bacilli, generally of the bovine type. In regard to adhesions, I have found in many cases of violent infection of the peritoneum an exudate which prevents adhesion or agglutination. I would lay stress on the culture test at the time of operation to prove whether the tuberculous infection is due to bovine or the human type.

Dr. C. L. Hall, Kansas City, Mo.: I do not arise so much to discuss the paper as to emphasize the point made by Dr. Truesdale in the discussion in regard to drainage, which, if it is in order, I would say applies to all abdominal drainage. It is now many years since I have introduced gauze of any description into the peritoneal cavity, and I find simply the folding of a part of a rubber glove or a soft rubber tissue so as to make a vent in the abdomen answers every purpose. Anything else becames a stench and a disagreeable feature. I introduce rubber tubage, soft as a rubber glove, and it will answer the results. I feel if the vent is made in the abdomen the natural peristalsis of the bowel—the breathing and extension of the diaphragm—will promote drainage.

Dr. E. E. Montgomery, Philadelphia: I should like to emphasize the importance of microscopic investigation of all specimens removed. We are not able to determine, in cases of this character, what the pathogenic condition is unless such an investigation has been made, and it will reveal, not infrequently, that tuberculosis or other conditions existed when they were unsuspected. Four years ago, at the Los Angeles meeting I reported a case in which I had removed a mass from one side about the size of a walnut, and which was supposed at the time to be a fibroid of the fallopian tube. Investigation proved it to be a carcinoma. Remembering the opposite tube was somewhat enlarged at the time of operation, I immediately reopened this woman and removed the uterus and its other appendage. The investigation of the other tube disclosed tuberculosis; so that we had in the patient a malignant disease on one side and a tuberculous disease on the other. Extension of inflammation from the peritoneum to the tube, even though it may be closed, I think is possible.

In a patient on whom I operated some years ago, and removed fibroid growths, a tuberculous peritonitis was found on the left side of the pelvis. Good health followed for some time, when she developed distress in the bladder and was treated quite awhile for cystitis, for which she again came under observation. I found a thickening of the side of the pelvis which, from its situation, was evidently the ureter. Later I removed the left kidney and its ureter for extensive tuberculous degeneration of the kidney and the entire ureter which I attributed to the previous infection extending from the involved peritoneum. With regard to the removal of such a mass, in my judgment, it is quite important that the tube should be removed in patients in whom we recognize a tuberculous condition existing, even though the tube may be open, because of the possibility of extension of such inflammation; the fact that the patient has a tuberculous disease makes it less desirable in her case that she should give birth to progeny than an individual in good health; so, it would seem wise in cases of tuberculous infection of the ovaries that they should be removed.

DR. S. M. D. CLARK, New Orleans: Dr. Taylor touched a very significant point when he referred to the importance of routine examination of specimens. Five or six years ago, I recall when my specimens were sent to the general pathologic department that the percentage of tuberculosis in these cases was not as high as usually found in other clinics. Since adopting the dual method of not only using the regular pathologic service, but in addition employing one especially interested in pelvic pathology, the finding of tuberculosis has notably increased and the percentage has materially risen. I have always looked on the tubes and appendix as having a selective affinity for tuberculosis, and in the great bulk of cases the primary abdominal focus was in these structures. The splendid work in this field of Murphy and Mayo is most striking; therefore, when dealing with tuberculous peritonitis, the first regions to be explored are the tubes and appendix, believing that in their removal a larger percentage of cures will follow. For the past eight months when finding a tuberculous endometrium, I have removed the tubes only and find that the endometrium returns to normal, proving that in nearly all cases the disease of the endometrium is secondary to the tubal disease.

DR. HOWARD C. TAYLOR, New York: It is practically impossible to determine in any case whether the tube or the peritoneum was primarily affected. The cases reported by Krönig, in which one tube after removal was demonstrated microscopically to be tuberculous, and in which the remaining tube was probably tuberculous, demonstrates that a tuberculous peritonitis certainly does not always follow a tuberculous salpingitis. Conversely, the fact that tuberculous salpingitis is usually bilateral is in favor of the salpingitis being secondary to a peritonitis and not the result of a hematogenous infection. I am glad so many have spoken of the necessity of examining every tube removed. It has become more or less common if a woman shortly after marriage starts up an inflammatory condition in the pelvis, at once to draw the conclusion that there is a gonorrheal infection. I think that this is not correct, and that the true explanation is that there is an acute exacerbation of an old tuberculous lesion.

THE APPLICATION OF THE VARIOUS THEORIES IN THE MANAGEMENT OF PERITONITIS

WILLIAM D. HAGGARD, M.D.

Fellow of the American College of Surgeons; Professor of Surgery and
Clinical Surgery at Vanderbilt University; Surgeon to
St. Thomas Hospital; Visiting Surgeon to
Vanderbilt and City Hospitals

NASHVILLE, TENN.

In spite of nearly three decades of effort in the prophylaxis of peritonitis there are yet, even in cases that should be prevented, many examples of this disease that under any method of treatment still yield a very high mortality. While this has been greatly curtailed, and betterment in early recognition and efficient treatment is constant, there have been several additions to the plans of management which are worthy of consideration and application.

The beginning of the operative treatment of this disease yielded a frightful death rate, because we were as pioneers in its handling, and while our methods have been vastly enhanced in point of effectiveness, the disease is still as formidable as ever. At the Russian Congress of Surgeons in 1913 there was reported a mortality of 60.9 per cent. in 758 cases of the various forms of peritonitis. In cases occurring after forty-eight hours the death rate was 78 per cent. It is obvious that these statistics are appalling. Without any invidious criticism of our confrères, it is incontrovertible that in America we have nothing near so desperate a mortality, and yet our results are far from being ideal.

Next to the introduction of operative intervention for the elimination of the focus of peritoneal infection, the greatest adjunct in its treatment is the recognition

of the forces at work in Nature's behalf and their conservation. It has been notorious that the most inopportune time for intervention is the period too late to
anticipate the widespread invasion of the peritoneum
and too early to allow for the benefits of the effort
which Nature puts forth in her own behalf. The peritoneum is wonderfully efficient in protecting itself and
destroying its invaders. The results of operation in
the very early hours of the disease are most brilliant.
Likewise in the terminal stages, as the result of the
successful efforts at localization with the formation of
localized abscess, the surgical task is greatly simplified
and the results pleasing. In the interim when the
battle wages, especially on the third, fourth and fifth
days of the disease, our procedures are perilous, and
herein lies the great difficulty of decision. The active
group of surgeons immediately preceding our own
time call attention to this fact. Cartledge in 1900 was
among the first to draw attention to the undesirability
of operating in peritonitis of appendiceal origin, in
the third, fourth and fifth days, and yet operation was
probably better than the purely nonoperative measures
of that time.

It remained for Ochsner, with his searching inquiry
and bold persistence, to point out a way by which
these bad cases could be converted into safer risks.
His methods are well known. In the beginning
they were misunderstood by the medical man, who
disregarded the first rule laid down by him, to operate
in all cases of appendicitis in the first thirty-six hours
when a competent surgeon was available. Moreover,
his teachings at first were violently opposed by the
surgical side, who realized the great need for therapy
of some sort for the ravages of peritonitis. They
were unmindful of the successful issue of many apparently very bad cases by Nature's efforts. We were
constantly seeing walled-off abscesses in the peritoneum, which were uniformly evacuated with success,
without taking into consideration how it was encom-

passed by Nature and how we might aid it. Ochsner
taught us that absolute quietude of the patient, and
inhibition of peristalsis was the desideratum. Nearly
everybody learned the starvation feature but disregarded the underlying principles, and still persisted in
the mischievous and often murderous efforts at purgation. At present, ten years after Ochsner's plan was
given to us, it is a frequent and sad experience to see
widely diffused peritonitis as the result of purgation
plus delay. The latter is bad enough, but the lesser
evil.

Ochsner says he has never seen a death from peritonitis (I presume he means of appendiceal origin)
when no food or purgatives were given from the start.
That ideal condition is rarely obtainable. Any practitioner, sufficiently versed in the pathology and needs
of peritonitic cases, would recognize the wisdom of
very early surgical relief. When neither are appreciated by him, the surgeon has to choose, on the one
hand, between the late institution of the Ochsner plan,
when the harm from the infraction of its three fundamentals, early operation, absence of food, and withholding purgation has actually accrued, and, on the
other hand, the risk incurred by operation. With the
perfected modern operation and the valuable postoperative auxiliary methods of after-treatment, most surgeons under these circumstances employ operative
measures.

Thus in 516 cases of appendicitis, of all grades of
severity, operated in the last four years, with 13 operative deaths, 2.5 per cent., I declined only 4 cases, too
desperate for operation, which, added to the operative
mortality, make 17 deaths, or 3.2 per cent.

Deaver[1] has lately shown the devastating effects of
purgation. He asserts that purgation is more deadly
than the scalpel, and analyzes seventy-nine cases with
a history of purgation and found in all save two, at

---

1. Deaver: Internat. Clin., iii, Series 22, p. 242.

the time of operation for appendicitis, that the organ was either perforated, gangrenous, or surrounded by an abscess. Of seven deaths in his series, five patients had been purged, and of those who had been drastically purged, nearly all showed a very severe type of disease. The purge in peritonitis is the submarine to Nature's allies.

The value of gastric lavage, before and after operation in peritonitis, is incontrovertible. The removal of quantities of decomposed food, or even bile with the mysterious poison which seems to emanate from the duodenum, is very essential. In its employment, however, one should not neglect to cocainize the pharynx. This gastric lavage, if attended by great resistance, straining and vomiting, while intended to be beneficial, is about as harmful as food or purgation in causing movements of viscera and dissemination of the infecting material.

All surgeons are agreed that in the advanced cases of peritonitis, when the patient shows a clammy blue skin, extremely rapid pulse, low or subnormal temperature, with great distention, a motionless abdomen, low white cell count or leukopenia, that operation is practically useless. Patients in cases of less severity may recover with gentle and skilful interference. It is not to be denied, however, that interference at an inopportune time sometimes brings disaster, when the utilization of the Ochsner principles, plus deep morphinization, might have availed. It is a common experience with fifth and sixth day cases, before the complete walling off has taken place, that when infection is at its zenith and the resistance of the patient has not yet overcome it, particularly when the condition is very grave, operation in all probability would prove fatal, and yet with these rational measures improvement is manifest and in a few days the abscess becomes encapsulated and can be cured by simple incision and drainage.

Page,[2] in a thoughtful article with reference to the localized form of peritonitis, says it is very definitely shown that opening a local abscess and draining without crossing the peritoneum is attended with a considerable death rate. He has advanced the idea of simply opening the abdomen, and if the abscess is not adherent to the abdominal wall, but is still effectively walled off, not to interfere with the abscess at all. He simply inserts a medium-sized cigaret drain to the outer side of the abscess cavity, and says in a very considerable number the inflammatory swelling subsides without any pus appearing.

In the event the temperature does not subside and the pain continues, he removes the tube after a few days, and under gas inserts a finger along the tract of the drainage tube and breaks into the abscess and drains it. It is obvious that a badly situated abscess is thus rendered extraperitoneal in its evacuation. He has by this conservative method treated nineteen localized abscesses with absolutely no deaths, as contrasted to three deaths in twenty-five cases treated by the ordinary method at St. Thomas Hospital in London.

Contrasted to this plan, Knott[3] has urged the evacuation of all localized abscesses, after having sequestrated the outlying peritoneum, removing the appendix in every instance and draining the pelvis with gauze in a split rubber tube. He reports 501 cases with a mortality of 1.2 per cent. This practice has been employed more and more in this country, and is now almost the routine plan unless the localized abscess is ancient — 10 to 14 days — and adherent to the abdominal wall. In such cases I stop with evacuation and drainage, and do not search for the appendix.

In every case of peritonitis, whether localized or not, one should never fail to explore the pelvis with a long

2. Page: Brit. Med. Jour., Nov. 1, 1914.
3. Knott, Van Buren: The Removal of the Appendix in All Cases of Appendicitis with Localized Abscess, The Journal A. M. A., March 28, 1914, p. 1004.

glass catheter as a capillary tube, a small sponge on holder, or a suprapubic incision if the original incision or focus has been in the upper abdomen. Often large quantities of more or less infected fluid will well up.

The knowledge of the danger zones in peritonitis, the greatest of which has been shown to be the upper abdomen and the least vulnerable the pelvis, led Fowler to suggest the upright position which has since caused his name to be associated with the great improvement in the treatment of this disease. Its wide adaptation has been one of the signal advances.

Murphy's addition to the principles of early operation, minimum interference (compatible with) rapid and efficient work, was the instillation of large quantities of salt solution through the rectum. It restores body fluids, dilutes toxins in the blood current, causes a great transudation of serum into the peritoneum, irrigates it with its bacterins, and helps manufacture lymph for trench warfare around the focus of infection. Its technic, however, while not in the purview of this paper, needs to be very actively gaged to insure results. As a maximum, 18 pints should be administered in twenty-four hours. When it is not retained, Murphy says it is the fault of the method of administration.

If it is necessary to obtain the anatomic and physiologic rest by withholding food, cathartics, gastric lavage and rectal infusion, was the old theory of Alonzo Clark — the use of large quantities of opium to absolutely inhibit peristalsis — so very erroneous? When the real pathology was uncovered surgically, this theory was thought to be exploded.

Recently Crile, in advancing the fascinating kinetic theory of peritonitis, has in effect drawn our attention to the very great value of deep morphinization to insulate the patient from the fatal dissipation of his energy in fighting his disease.

He has shown that the lethal results of peritonitis are due to the great exhaustion with its destructive

action on the great organs, that is, the brain, the liver
and the adrenals.   This results from the enforced
transformation of potential into kinetic energy used
in defense.   All of the local and general symptoms
are Nature's combative response to the infection.   The
pain compels the patient to assume a "box-like rigidity."   The anorexia, vomiting and obstipation prevent
ingestion and the dissemination of infection by peristalsis.   The temperature burns up the protein com-
pounds of infection.   The distention of paresis, the
exudation of lymph, the gluing of viscera together, are
efforts at walling off infectious areas or products.
All these symptoms, therefore, are really wonderful,
automatic and often successful efforts at protection
and self-cure, but they require great expenditures of
kinetic energy.   Can we protect the individual from
this loss of energy while the "offensive movement" of
phagocytosis continues?   If the patient were asleep
and oblivious to the conflict that was costing him
nothing in the output of energy, he would be thus
aided and abetted while his forces overcame the infection.   This can be greatly promoted in the severest
cases that cannot be handled in the usual way by
keeping the individual deeply narcotized with morphin
after operation.   The respirations should be held down
to 12 or 14 per minute.   I have employed this method
in addition to the usual plans after operation in three
recent cases of general suppurative peritonitis with two
recoveries, neither of which I believe would have
resulted without the mental, physical and cellular
immobility of the protective influence of deep narcotization.

The restoration of energy can be kept up by the
introduction of large quantities of fluid, by the seeping
method of Murphy.   Plain water as advocated by
Trout can be used or it can be impregnated with salt,
glucose for nourishment, or sodium bicarbonate to
antidote acidosis.   By the anoci method Crile has
been able to reduce his deaths to only two in 391 cases

of acute appendicitis, with and without peritonitis, with the addition of narcotization in the very severe cases.

In general diffuse, suppurative peritonitis, the mortality under any method of treatment is staggering. It is not so much the impotence of our various plans of treatment, as the delay in employing them. Everything depends on promptitude. It is profitless to consider the cases of this class statistically as the time limit, virulence and extent of involvement vary so widely. One can never know whether the entire peritoneal membrane is implicated or not. If it is, and sufficient delay has occurred to bring this about, then an enormous death rate is inevitable under any and all known methods of treatment. All cases of peritonitis from perforation of stomach, duodenum, or other hollow viscera by gunshot or stab wounds, imperatively require operation within the first eight hours if possible. I have recently operated successfully at the end of eighteen hours, following a perforated duodenal ulcer, in a man of 56 who had been transported a considerable distance, but it is incontrovertible that the mortality rises with amazing rapidity with each hour intervening before operation.

The opportunities for the improvement in the results of peritonitis have never been more satisfactory. Early recognition of its causes is becoming more universal, although it may be admitted that whenever a case of advanced peritonitis, particularly from the appendix, has to be dealt with, it is proof of faulty management up to that time.

The most essential treatment, therefore, with or without operation, is an absolute prohibition of anything whatsoever by mouth, with immediate preparation for operative relief when possible. When for any reason this cannot be done the continuance of this principle with the addition of deep morphinization are the most dependable methods. After operation drainage by the glass tube suprapubically and the employment of the upright posture and proctoclysis is well nigh routine.

The various theories herein considered can be judicially employed for the varying manifestations of peritonitis, and by a judicious combination of the plans briefly referred to in this paper and the perfection of the technic of each, it is believed that the prevalence of peritonitis by surgical prophylaxis can be greatly reduced, and the percentage of cures when its progress has not been immediately prevented can be very appreciably augmented.

184 Eighth Avenue North.

ABSTRACT OF DISCUSSION

DR. WILLIAM B. BRINSMADE, Brooklyn: Let me call to mind the picture you have seen so often. A poor patient is seen, generally late at night; the lips are pale, the abdomen is distended, the pulse weak, the respiration labored; as you lift the covering the odor of flaxseed or turpentine, chloroform or some liniment greets your nostrils. As you put your hand on the abdomen, the patient flinches and perhaps brings up a few ounces of bile-stained fluid. Then comes the history of an acute onset—pain, vomiting, and gradually increasing constipation. The treatment has consisted of salts, castor oil, more salts, more oil, soapsuds enemas, turpentine enemas, alum enemas—and you are told that everything has been tried for three days and nothing has done any good, and therefore the salvage corps has been called on in the shape of a surgeon. Inquiry develops that the poor patient has had something done to her hourly, and has had no sleep for two or three days. Such a case demands an operation in the early stage; after forty-eight hours of a progressive invasion, operation is positively contra-indicated. If there is a chance for the poor soul it lies in rest—rest for the stomach and bowels, rest for the body, rest for the brain, and this can be best attained by a large dose of morphin and gastric lavage. If the fates are with her, the patient may recover sufficiently to undergo the indicated surgical interference. If the surgeon operates, she will, in ninety-nine cases out of a hundred, pass on to the land from which there is no returning. Peritonitis is not a primary disease and of course should not be allowed to occur, but it does occur and always will. The time to operate and the method of operation are questions of the wisest judgment, which the surgeon is ever called on to exercise. If the patient can stand the burden of an operation, an incision over the original focus of disease with drainage, and an added suprapubic drain will fill the immediate requirements. Rectal and vaginal examinations will occasionally indicate the route for drainage of the pelvis.

DR. JOHN O. POLAK, Brooklyn: I desire to call attention to the importance of the application of part of Dr. Haggard's paper to the gynecologic and puerperal forms of peritonitis. If there is one class of peritoneal involvement that needs Ochsnerism, it is the class that follows the abortion or the exacerbated gonorrheal infection or a puerperal infection, for there is no class with which operative procedure is fraught with such mortality, morbidity and anatomic sacrifice. The principle which I lay down for the practitioner to follow is that where there is peritoneal irritation, particularly when there is a history of pelvic origin, that case is not to be treated with salts and fed— but to have absolute starvation and morphin and the Fowler position, and I go further; I believe these pelvic cases do better if we omit the Murphy drip and use a 2 per cent. glucose solution by hypodermoclysis. We have carried these patients for many days. Serious distention, due to the paresis, will subside, the tongue be kept moist, and the vomiting cease. Lavage, morphin, hypodermoclysis, the Fowler position and leaving these patients alone is the general plan. When we operate, we operate for a definite pus formation. Where there is an exudate we wait and never operate until the case falls within the rule Simpson has laid down; i. e., the temperature has remained normal for a long time—he puts it three weeks in the classical cases— when the exudate has disappeared and the examination does not increase and cause an exacerbation of the temperature or exudate and when the leukocyte count has remained below eleven thousand.

DR. EDWARD REYNOLDS, Boston: I wish to speak of certain points in the technic of the operative management of the walled-off abdomen. Everyone agrees that when this class of abdomen can be gotten at through the vagina without opening uninfected peritoneum above, that is preferable. But when that is not possible one must open from above. First and foremost in importance is quick, brief, gentle operation. If one opens and finds that one is well away from the walled off part, instant, thorough walling-off is required, and if one opens within the adhesions, walling off from the start with gauze, that at least no more peritoneum may be infected. When one gets down to the thickened adhesions behind which we know the pus lies, use a little fresh, separate gauze, before the finger goes through the adhesions and opens the actual pus cavity, that pus may be protected even from the walling off gauze. Follow by gentle evacuation, drainage, and the removing of the gauze in actual contact with the pus, without disturbing the walling off of the more distant peritoneum. I have had the greatest satisfaction since I have begun to sop out the infected area with sponges dripping with alcohol, cleansing the peritoneum as I would any other thing. Of course sop out the cavity, if it is possible, and then use iodin on the infected surfaces. The drainage should be placed in situ before the disinfection. The whole procedure should be completed as rapidly and gently as possible. I have had a better percentage of recovery since I began the fearless application of alcohol to the whole infected area and tincture of iodin to the actually traumatized area in those infected cases.

Dr. J. B. DeLee, Chicago: Diagnosis is important. There is a distinct difference in the mortality of surgical peritonitis and obstetric peritonitis. Most cases of appendicitis get well without operation. Immediate drainage is not advised. The abscess should be allowed to form and can be opened later when the mortality is lower. On the other hand, puerperal peritonitis after a full term labor has a very high mortality and I was hoping that Dr. Haggard would present some successful method of treating these patients. I have tried all the methods that Dr. Haggard has so ably presented. The women die in spite of all you do in general puerperal peritonitis.

The borderline cases of peritonitis offer a better prognosis. After abortions and when the inflammation is limited to the pelvis, a more expectant plan of treatment is to be recommended. The Fowler position, the withholding of food for two or three days, large doses of opium—I prefer opium as it has a more sedative effect. When localization begins the longer the operation is postponed the better. As long as there is a continuous fever it is wise to keep out. There are cases in which an operation in the early stages of puerperal peritonitis may be indicated.

I would like to mention the facility with which the abdomen may be opened. You can turn the patient across the bed, insert a speculum and open the culdesac; a few injections of novocain around the cervix will make the operation as painless as the filling of a tooth. The abdomen may be opened very simply. The patient does not have to be taken out of bed; painting the skin with iodin, novocain is injected along the line of incision and in five or six minutes the operation is completed.

Dr. H. O. Pantzer, Indianapolis: On opening the abdomen and finding free fluid, nonodorous, beside an abscess distinctly foul, I have learned such a condition to indicate a favorable prognosis. The observation first leading up to this was in a child 6 months old, with a general peritonitis in connection with a gangrenous appendicitis. The abdomen was full of purulent nonodorous fluid. The abscess contained about 45 c.c. of a thick, creamy, very foul pus. The child made an uneventful and speedy recovery. This observation was repeatedly verified in similar cases during the nine years since then, and I have come to regard this sign as of real prognostic value. One point in regard to therapy. Given a case which is drifting rapidly toward death, as indicated by dryness of skin, foulness and dryness of tongue, coma, etc., and which indicates in itself a toxemia which the glands can no longer cope with, here large doses of sodium salicylate—30 or even 60 grains at a dose—are of eminent usefulness. Given by rectum, with one pint of water and a few drops of camphor every four hours, this medication will often do wonders.

RELATIVE FREQUENCY OF ECTOPIC GESTATION

ALFRED BAKER SPALDING, A.B., M.D.

Professor of Obstetrics and Gynecology, Leland Stanford Junior
University, School of Medicine

SAN FRANCISCO

Why an impregnated ovum should implant and develop outside the uterus so relatively frequently in the human species and fail to do so in lower animals is a question the answer to which has been sought through investigation by clinicians and laboratory workers for a great many years. Clinicians agree that ectopic gestation is a frequent abnormality of early pregnancy but vary in their estimates of frequency depending on whether their clinical experience has been gained as a necropsy surgeon, a gynecologist, an obstetrician or a general practitioner. The large number of case reports indicate the frequency with which this condition is met by surgeons, but is too irrelevant to be of aid in discussing the subject statistically. In this paper, a statistical study of a definite number of patients will be made in order to estimate the relative frequency of ectopic gestation to disease in general, to women's disease, to pregnancy and to abortion. The small material presented makes the importance of the subject the sole excuse for presuming to answer these difficult questions.

The necropsy surgeon reports that he frequently meets ectopic gestation because sudden death associated with such a condition requires his services to satisfy the demands of the law. The gynecologist considers ectopic pregnancy a frequent condition because he does not take into account the many ordinary conditions which the man in general practice has treated before referring to him the patient with ectopic pregnancy. The obstetrician considers ectopic gestation a relatively rare condition because, through lack of understanding, the laity are prone to come to him only after the first three dangerous months of pregnancy are passed. It is an odd experience that a general practitioner may encounter several ectopic pregnancies quite close together and then practice for some time without meeting a case.

Formad,[1] who was a coroner's physician in Philadelphia, in 3,500 routine necropsies, found thirty-five deaths from ectopic pregnancy. Michel[2] has reported twenty-six cases of ectopic gestation in 6,000 gynecologic conditions, while Hartz[3] reports 3.4 per cent. of ectopic pregnancy in 1,700 specimens examined in the gynecologic laboratory at Jefferson and St. Joseph's hospitals in Philadelphia. Hennig[4] stated some years ago that the directors of even large obstetric institutions might never encounter a case.

Although ectopic gestation is discussed in textbooks on obstetrics, no modern obstetrician has, to my knowledge, ventured an opinion of its frequency based on his personal experience. My own experience has been that for ten years, while limiting my practice to obstetrics, I did not treat a case of ectopic pregnancy in private or clinic work, but during the last three years while combining gynecology with obstetrics, I have operated on thirteen clinic patients and on seven private patients for this condition. The clinic cases form the basis for this paper as they were encountered at fairly regular intervals in a comparatively large number of patients.

From July 1, 1912, to May 1, 1915 (the time of writing), 36,668 patients have registered in the out-

1. From an unpublished communication by Ellice McDonald.
2. Michel: Fortschr. d. Med., 1914, No. 23, p. 637.
3. Hartz: Am. Jour. Obst., 1915, lxxi, 601.
4. Hennig: Die Krankheiter der Erleiter und die Tubenschwangerschaft, Stuttgart, 1876.

patient clinics of the Leland Stanford University, School of Medicine. Of this number, 2,955 have been treated in the women's clinic. In the clinic, fairly extensive histories of the patients were taken and a careful pelvic examination made, as well as considerable routine laboratory work started. A presumptive clinical diagnosis was entered on the history as soon as conditions justified such procedure. These facts are mentioned because often the diagnosis of early pregnancy is impossible, and because some patients, so soon as that diagnosis is made, fail to report to the clinic. Many cases of pregnancy abort or are aborted after leaving the clinic, and possibly some cases of ectopic gestation are overlooked. Taking these facts into consideration, it is interesting to note that of the 2,955 patients registered in the women's clinic, 554 were operated on for various gynecologic conditions. Of these, 353 were curetted and the curettings, together with the associated pathology, were studied in the laboratory for obstetrics and gynecology.

From these specimens there have been made seventy-three laboratory diagnoses of incomplete abortion and thriteen diagnoses of ectopic pregnancy, 1,225 of the 2,955 patients were confined by the clinic at or near term, which makes a total of 1,311 known pregnancies and 468 patients operated on who were known not to be pregnant.

The remaining group of 1,176 patients who did not enter the hospital includes undoubtedly some cases of pregnancy, but is composed largely of nonpregnant patients such as come to all clinics for treatment of minor gynecologic ailments, as well as patients past the childbearing period, and a few children. The statistical work with this group is not as accurate as with the hospital group and the proportion of pregnant to nonpregnant patients can be estimated only roughly. Still it is important to include with the known pregnancies a fair number of these doubtful cases. For ten years, I have recorded annually the percentage of pregnant

CLINICAL SUMMARY OF ETIOLOGIC CONDITIONS IN ECTOPIC GESTATION

Case	Age	Grav.	Para	Abortions, Induced	Abortions, Spontaneous	Gonorrhea	Last Pregnancy, Yrs.	Leukocytosis 10,000+	H. Per Cent, 60 or Lower	Tube Rupt.	Tube Unrupt.	Tube Abor. Comp.	Tube Abor. Incomp.	Clinical Diagnosis	Salpingitis Microscopic	Tube Decidua	Fetus Present	Mortality, Fetus	Mortality, Mother
1	25	4i	ii	0	1	+	5	~	~	:	:	:	+	Pelvic abscess	+	—	—	+	—
2*	35	vii	ii	▶	0	+	6	+	~	:	:	+	:	Salpingo-oophoritis	+	+	—	+	—
3	30	iii	1	0	1	—	7	—	+	+	:	:	:	Ectopic	+	—	—	+	—
4	35	iii	n	1	0	—	5	—	—	:	:	:	+	Ectopic ?	—	—	—	+	—
5	28	ii	1	1	0	—	11	+	~	:	:	:	+	Pelvic abscess	+	+	+	+	—
6	28	ii	0	1	0	+	12	+	+	+	:	:	:	Appendicitis	—	+	—	+	—
7	29	ii	0	0	1	—	2	+	+	+	:	:	:	Salpingitis	+	+	+	+	—
8	34	i	0	0	1	—	7	+	—	:	:	:	+	Pelvic abscess	+	—	—	+	—
9	40	ix	0	0	0	—	0	+	+	:	+	:	:	Uterus	+	+	+	+	—
10	21	i	▶	|||	0	—	1	~	+	+	:	:	:	stone	+		—	+	—
11	24	iii	0	0	0	+	0	+			+	+	:	:	:	?	+	+	—	+	—
12	29	iii	0	0	0	—	19	+	+	:	+	:	+	Incomplete abortion	—	+	—	+	—
13		iii	1	0	1	—	8	~	+	:	+	:	:	Incomplete abortion	—	+	+	#	—
Aver.	30	III	1	..	..	..	6	80%	60%	..	..	..	..		60%	40%	30%	100%	0
Total	..	43	14	11	5	4	..	..	..	5	2	1	5						

* At operation there was found a leather-like fetus 8 cm. long compressed between a pus tube and the fibrous uterus. The patient survived a tube abortion, which undoubtedly occurred six years ago, associated with an attempted criminal abortion.

† In the laboratory there was found a hematosalpinx containing cartilage cells which, with the history, gave evidence that the patient survived an ectopic pregnancy four years ago, mistaking the conditions for a spontaneous abortion.

: Ectopic pregnancy.   ‖ Left tube and ovary removed.

Fetus alive at time of operation.   ¶ On hospital entrance slip.

patients that have failed to return to the San Francisco maternity clinic for confinement, and have found that, on the average, 25 per cent. of the applicants do so fail to return. Applying this experience to the present clinical material, 393 of the 1,176 doubtful cases, or 30 per cent. of the number of confinements, have been grouped with the known pregnancies, making a total of 1,704 pregnancies, and 783 have been grouped with the operated patients, making a total of 1,251 nonpregnant patients.

From these figures, it will be seen that we have met ectopic gestation thirteen times in 36,668 patients or once in 2,820 cases of illness such as a general practitioner would encounter in a practice covering the diseases of men, women and children. Thirteen cases of ectopic gestation among 2,955 women with pelvic symptoms, or once in 227 cases such as come to the specialist; and thirteen cases of ectopic gestation among 1,704 cases of pregnancy, or once in each 131 pregnancies!

Considering the pathologic diagnoses which have been made in the laboratory, it is seen that 86, or 5.33 per cent. of the pregnant patients were sent into the hospital because of bleeding, and were curetted. A study of these curettements has shown that thirteen of the 86 patients, or nearly 17 per cent. of possible abortions, were flowing because they were suffering with a misplaced pregnancy.

This does not indicate the relative frequency of abortion to pregnancy, which has been estimated by Taussig[5] as high as one abortion to every 2.3 labors, but will, I believe, call attention to the possibility of confusing ectopic gestation with incomplete abortion and should put the general practitioner on his guard when treating such cases.

Albucasis,[6] an Arabian surgeon of the eleventh century, is said to have first described ectopic pregnancy. For generations the etiology of the condition was little

5. Taussig: Prevention and Treatment of Abortion, St. Louis, 1910.
6. Aboulcassem Khalaf ben Abbas Ezzahraony.

understood, but gradually the idea prevailed that, in many cases at least, an inflammatory condition of the adnexa was the predisposing cause.

Dr. William Campbell[7] accumulated these data and published a monograph which later formed the basis of Parry's[8] work and to whom Lawson Tait[9] gives great credit in discussing the subject.

Lawson Tait[9] said, "I believe it to be more than likely that the real cause of this accident is the coincidence of a set of circumstances the most important of which is the destruction or insufficiency of the ciliary movement." Since Tait made this statement, however investigators have shown that often the cilia are not destroyed. Moreover, the condition of round-cell infiltration, of destruction of the surface epithelium, of agglutination of the septa of the tubes, of edema and fibrosis, which are frequently present in the ectopic tube, are stated by some pathologists to depend on the condition of the existing pregnancy or the recent rupture of the tube rather than a preexisting inflammation. Careful sections of the tubes also show that in some cases the ovum has lodged in a blind passage supposed to be a congenital abnormality.

Webster[10] states that the ovum always imbeds in müllerian tissue and Huffman,[11] on theoretic considerations, carries his idea farther by stating that the ovum always imbeds, in cases of ectopic pregnancy, in anomalous imbedding areas. While these theories are attractive, they lead away from the clinical idea of inflammation and tend to place the predisposing cause of the condition on an unchangeable hereditary basis rather than on the basis of previous inflammatory affections which are preventable. Moreover, it should

7. Campbell, William: A Memoir on Extra Uterine Gestation, Edinburgh, 1842.

8. Parry: Extra Uterine Pregnancy: Its Causes, Species, Pathological Anatomy, Clinical History, Diagnosis, Prognosis and Treatment, Philadelphia, H. C. Lea, 1876.

9. Tait, R. Lawson: Diseases of Women, Philadelphia, Lea, 1879.

10. Webster: Study of a Specimen of Ovarian Pregnancy, Am. Jour. Obst., 1904. L. 28.

11. Huffman, Otto V.: A Theory of the Cause of Ectopic Pregnancy, THE JOURNAL A. M. A., Dec. 13, 1913, p. 2130.

not be forgotten that decidual reaction of early pregnancy has been noted in the tissues of practically all the organs of the lower abdomen, including the omentum and the appendix.[12] Leo Loeb[13] recently concludes that guinea-pigs do not have ectopic pregnancy because it is impossible to create in them a decidual reaction outside the uterus. One reason for the frequency of ectopic gestation in human beings undoubtedly depends on the ability of the tissues into which the ovum penetrates to develop decidua, which affords the ovum an adequate soil for development, but this does not eliminate the fact that pelvic inflammations often result in deformities of the tubes, which causes the ovum not infrequently to imbed outside the uterus.

A clinical summary of the cases here reported is presented in chart form and from this it will be seen that the average age, the multigravida, the number of preceding induced and spontaneous abortions as well as attacks of gonorrhea, the period of relative sterility and the microscopic findings all point strongly to the clinical idea of Tait that many of the cases of ectopic gestation trace their etiology to a preceding pelvic infection. It might be added that gonorrhea plays the minor rôle, and that abortion, associated as it so often is with a more or less noticeable attack of salpingitis, is the major predisposing cause for this frequent, dangerous anomaly of pregnancy.

CONCLUSIONS

From a statistical study of 36,668 clinic patients, the relative frequency of ectopic pregnancy is estimated as follows:

General practice..................Once in 2,820 cases
Gynecology ....Once in   227 cases
Pregnancy ....Once in   131 cases
Early pregnancy with hemorrhage
    (necessitating curettement)......Once in   7 cases
Lane Hospital.

---

12. Meyer, R.: Ektopiche Decidua, Ztschr. f. Geburtsh. u. Gynäk., 1914, lxxv, 760.
13. Loeb, Leo.: Tr. Soc. Exper. Biol. and Med., 1913, xi.

ABSTRACT OF DISCUSSION

Dr. Joseph B. De Lee, Chicago: Ectopic gestation occurs not infrequently in the lower animals, the horse especially, the cow and others. I know an interesting case in a house dog, running for six or eight weeks with symptoms of peritonitis. A roentgenogram disclosed the location of the fetus, an operation was performed, and a happy recovery made. As to the frequency of ectopic gestation, in my early years, in my hospital services everything except the actual delivery of a baby was assigned to the surgeon or to the gynecologist, and therefore, the obstetrician did not get the cases. He was considered perhaps one or two degrees better than a midwife, and of a different sex. This was the only distinction that I could learn. But as I began to assert my rights, and obtained all the obstetric cases, I found that the frequency of extrauterine pregnancy was increased. Perhaps we are losing sight of the point that so-called colics shortly after marriage, sometimes diagnosed as appendicitis, are not infrequently ectopic gestation aborting through the tube. You all know prostitutes' or actress' colic, and occasionally you hear of an actress being carried off the stage in a fainting condition. These are frequently cases aborting through the fallopian tube, and if properly diagnosed would increase the number of ectopic gestations which occur.

Dr. Alfred B. Spalding, San Francisco: I am not very much of a veterinarian and cannot dispute the point with Dr. DeLee about the ectopics occurring in the lower animals, but a great deal of work along this line has been done by others and many of the supposed cases of the ectopics in lower animals have been considered to be due to rupture of the uterus and to a secondary implantation of the ovum in the abdominal cavity.

Also the relation of the tube to the double uterus in the lower animals is different from that found in the human being. Loeb's work was on guinea-pigs. He found that it was impossible to make them have an ectopic pregnancy by any mechanical or experimental means, and they are not supposed to have an ectopic from natural causes. He was able in one case to get a supposed ectopic from a suspected rupture in the tube, which later was found to be a rupture of that part of the uterus which forms the connecting link between the two.

PROGNOSIS OF STERILITY

EDWARD REYNOLDS, M.D.
BOSTON

The treatment and more especially the operative treatment of sterility differs essentially from the treatment of ill health in that in the latter treatment is a matter of necessity, while in sterility it is frequently a matter of the patients' choice, of their readiness to submit to operation, or to perhaps tedious minor treatment, merely for the sake of future gain and happiness. For this reason an exact statement of the prognosis, of the degree to which success can be expected in the individual case, is of perhaps greater importance than in any other branch of surgery.

The importance of this point and the fact that the subject of sterility is so complex that a full review of even one phase of it can be with difficulty compressed within so short a space, is the reason that this paper must neglect treatment and even the details of diagnosis in order to cover prognosis even roughly.[1]

At first sight the most obvious method of dealing with this subject would be by the statistical study of cases treated, but apart from the complexity of the subject and the enormous number of cases which would be necessary for an adequate study of the several classes of sterility, a statistical presentation is rendered useless by the practical fact that so soon as

---

1. The Causes and Treatment of Sterility in Women, Am. Jour. Med. Sc., August, 1907; Anteflexion of the Cervix and Spasm of the Uterine Ligaments in Relation to Retroversion, Dysmenorrhea and Sterility, Surg., Gynec. and Obst., July, 1911, p. 17; The Ultimate Results of the Conservative Surgery of the Ovaries, Surg., Gynec. and Obst., March, 1912, p. 255. Reynolds, Edward: The Theory and Practice of the Treatment of Sterility in women, THE JOURNAL A. M. A., Jan. 11, 1913, p. 93; Further Points on the Sterility of Women, ibid., Oct. 11, 1913, p. 1363.

one's study of sterility begins to bring him any considerable number of reference cases he sees an increasingly large proportion of cases which are on their face hopeless, the patients having traveled from place to place hoping against hope. The exclusion of these cases from his statistics would make them unconvincing and unreliable; their inclusion would make the results practically useless;[2] and further the only point which is of practical value is the attainment of an accurate prognosis in individual cases under the several classes of sterility, rather than a general statistical statement which would be of little value, and which, from the complexity of the subject, is all that could be obtained statistically from any number of actually observed cases which could today be collected.

In order to obtain a fair conception of the prognosis in any given case we must consider sterilities under a classification by causation, and must discuss, first, the :prognosis in each of these classes by itself, and. later, the prognosis in the many cases in which the sterility is due to more than one of these causes.

We may begin such a classification by dividing sterilities into those which are dependent on absence or inferior quality of the ovum, those which are the result of secretions of the genital tract which are destructive

---

2. As an illustration: After selecting, in preparation for this paper, a certain date from which a statistical investigation of personal cases should begin, and assembling all the cases seen since that date, the first seven cases showed the following conditions: Patient 1, both tubes and one ovary previously removed for tuberculosis. Patient 2, large pelvic masses after repeated operations for "peritonitis"; condition of husband unknown. Patient 3, both tubes enlarged; two previous abdominal operations; will contemplate nothing but minor treatment. Patient 4, ten years of gonorrheal salpingitis in first marriage; two previous operations; demanded operation in spite of bad prognosis; both tubes found ruined. Patient 5, aged 44; previous operation for genital tuberculosis; polypus of cervix; husband not accessible. Patient 6, husband partly impotent and refuses examination. Patient 7, anteflexion of the cervix, pinhole os, plastic operation; pregnant three months afterward. Here six hopeless cases were found before one was favorable. In nearly a hundred cases which were abstracted before the attempt was given up, the proportion of hopeless cases proved indeed to be smaller than this, but was still so high as to vitiate statistical conclusions. The percentage of hopeless cases was, moreover, found to increase in a general relation to the distance from which the patient had been referred, thus hinting in another way that a prognosis drawn statistically from such a list as this would not show fairly the prognosis of sterility in cases as the practitioner sees them, or as they exist in the community at large.

to either the ovum or spermatozoa, and finally those which are due to absence or inferior quality of the spermatozoa. In each of these classes we have cases · which are organic in nature, that is, due to local or anatomic abnormalities; and in each we see cases which are functional and due to abnormal constitutional conditions of the individual. We have, then, at least six classes to start from, and most of these must later be subdivided.

We are profoundly ignorant of the chemistry of the reproductive organs. We can then draw conclusions about the functional cases only from analogy with facts which have been more or less well established in the breeding of animals and by the very small amount of direct experimental work which has been done along lines bearing on sterility. After about three years of some personal study on this point in domestic fowls, and of inquiry among breeding farms devoted to animals it seems to be probably an established fact that, in animals, fertility is decreased both by undue obesity in either sex and by excessive overwork. There is also some reason to believe that conditions of life which produce marked nervous excitability decrease fertility in animals, and this must be remembered in connection with many of the conditions of civilized existence in the human race. We have, however, no knowledge of the mechanism by which such alterations of condition produce relative or compiete sterility in animals. We do not even know whether it is effected by decreased quality of the ova or spermatozoa of the individuals, or by alteration of the chemical composition of the fluids in which these gonads are immersed.

We know even less about this question in the human race. We however know a little more about this point in the human male than in the female on account of the ease with which the spermatozoa can be directly inspected and because of the impossibility of finding the ovum. We have direct evidence that in the human male an excess of mental work sometimes results in the disappearance of spermatozoa from his semen, and some direct evidence that an excess of fat may produce the same result. We have also probable clinical evidence that the excessive use of alcohol and perhaps the extremely excessive use of tobacco decrease the vitality of his spermatozoa even though they be still present and of normal appearance. We have absolutely no evidence concerning the effect of these general conditions on the ovum, and can only surmise that they may well have the same effect on the gonads of the female that they have on those of the male. This weakness of our knowledge of the functional conditions is necessarily a constant embarrassment in our interpretation of the importance of the organic or anatomic abnormalities which we detect in a given case.

In spite of this extremely unsatisfactory state of our scientific knowledge it is, however, possible to obtain very satisfactory practical results in the prognosis of individual cases by the assumption of the following working hypotheses:

1. When the spermatozoa are abundant in number, normal in form and appearance, furnished with long cilia and capable of rapid movement through the semen the male is satisfactorily fertile.

2. When normal spermatozoa are killed or lose vitality overrapidly in the secretions of the individual woman, the chemicophysiologic character of her secretions furnishes an effective cause of sterility.

3. The alterations in a secretion which make it fatal to the spermatozoon may be localized in the vagina, in the cervix, in the body of the uterus, or in one or both tubes; and any one of these alterations may exist with normal secretions above it; but an alteration in the secreting surface in any of these localities usually vitiates all the secretions below it, probably by their necessary admixture.

4. When the spermatozoa are observed to penetrate without apparent loss of vitality to the fundus of the uterus and to survive there for a normal length of time, deficient quality of the ova may be considered the probable cause of the sterility.

Throughout the management of every case of sterility it must be remembered that the failure is the failure not of one individual, but of a couple, and that the condition of both partners must be studied.

If these hypotheses are borne steadily in mind throughout the study of a case, and if the variations in the conditions which affect them are studied and restudied by all the methods which are now at our disposal, it becomes surprising to see how practically good a prognosis can usually be made in spite of our lack of exact physiology and chemistry, but, on the other hand, it is certainly true that so long as we labor under these defects of theoretic knowledge, a painstaking exactness in the observation of details will be the first prerequisite to success.

In the practical management of such a case the first step is the taking of a careful history, which should not be confined to the history of the sterility alone, but should follow every detail of the past health of both patients, since many sterilities are dependent on slight pathologic alterations in the genitals on which great light is often thrown by past symptomatology. The history and physical examination should also include a careful study of the general condition and especially of the nutrition and habits of life of both partners, such factors as obesity, emaciation, nervous debility, drug habits, sleeplessness from overwork, etc., in either partner, being all important. Furthermore, distasteful as the subject is, he who is to handle sterility successfully must acquire the art of obtaining full and accurately truthful histories of the sexual habits of the couple, with especial reference to any abnormalities, even if apparently minor, in either the sexual appetite, or the methods employed in the performance of coitus. There is certainly a steady percentage of cases in which these matters are all important. The next step in the management of the case from a practical standpoint is usually a careful examination of the genital tract of the woman step by step, remembering that minor abnormalities which are unimportant to health, that is, which create no symptoms of importance, are often abundantly competent to produce infertility. I constantly see cases which have been pronounced normal even by excellent gynecologists and in which the organs are normal from the standpoint of health, but in which there is nevertheless some minor abnormality which is perfectly evidently the cause of the sterility, as is often shown by the fact that when this is remedied impregnation occurs without further treatment. This examination must include study of the condition of the vagina, cervix, uterus (including the character of their secretions), tubes and ovaries, and it must be remembered that the detection of the minor abnormalities of the tubes and ovaries almost always requires an examination under anesthesia.

When all this has been gone through with sufficient care the surgeon should be in a position to estimate with considerable closeness both the anatomic and functional condition of the woman and should have an equally good estimate of the general functional condition of her husband.

In the majority of cases the next step should be a form of examination which has been lately given to the profession by the ingenuity of Dr. Max Huhner of New York, the microscopic examination of the spermatozoa in situ in the genitals of the woman, of which much will be said in the remainder of this paper, but dramatic and interesting as this test is, it must always be remembered that it can furnish at most only one element in our study of a case.

This test not only furnishes an examination of the man which is in most cases thoroughly satisfactory, but also enables us to check the conclusions previously arrived at as to the relative importance of anatomic and functional conditions by direct observation of much of the process of fertilization while actually in progress. Experience has, however, convinced me that this process of observation must, like so many other exact methods, be considered by the wise clinician as furnishing only one link in the chain of evidence. It is so interesting and dramatic that it is extremely easy to overestimate its value, and to be led by it to false conclusions, if we fail to consider its results in connection with those obtained by other methods of observation. If the conclusions arrived at by both methods are substantially in agreement, even to details, we may safely trust them. If the two methods yield different results we should distrust our conclusions, for we are then certainly not in a position to act until further study has reconciled their discrepancies. To pin our faith to either method will usually lead to false conclusions.

For the performance of the Huhner test we must ask to see the woman as soon as possible after coitus has taken place. She may come to the office for this examination, since it is only very exceptionally, if ever, that the vagina does not contain sufficient spermatozoa for this test even after she has walked about for some time. With a normal vaginal secretion the spermatozoa should show active motility in the vagina for about an hour and sometimes much longer, but if circumstances permit it is desirable that the patient should be seen within half an hour of coitus. A specimen of the vaginal mucus is taken by a sterile platinum wire from the culdesac, exposed by a speculum, and this examination may be repeated if desired, whenever convenience permits, until the spermatozoa are found to have lost their activity. A specimen of the cervical mucus is next obtained in the same way, after the surface of the cervix has first been carefully wiped clean of semen by the repeated use of cotton swabs (no antiseptic should be used). With a normal cervical secretion and a normal os a few spermatozoa will usually be found in the lower part of the cervical cavity almost immediately after coitus, but will appear there in larger numbers at the end of half an hour to an hour. They are never so numerous here as in the vagina, but under normal circumstances, at the end of an hour, there should be several actively moving spermatozoa in each slide from the cervical mucus. The greatest care should be used to avoid the infliction of any trauma in the examination of the cervical cavity, since over-thoroughness here may readily vitiate the use of the remaining portion of the test at that sitting.

When the cervical cavity has not been unduly disturbed, when the spermatozoa are of full vitality, and when the secretions of the woman are normal throughout, an examination of the secretions of the cavity of the uterine body should disclose the presence of a few actively motile spermatozoa in the uterine mucus at the end of from two to three or four hours. This examination must however be made with a specially devised syringe, since the platinum loop can neither be introduced with certainty to the fundus nor made to retain the uterine mucus during its withdrawal from the cervix. Even with the use of a syringe it is difficult to be absolutely sure that spermatozoa which are observed in the fluid withdrawn from the uterus are not due to an admixture from the cervix, but if the piston is not withdrawn until the tip of the syringe is well up in the uterine cavity, if the outside of the syringe is carefully wiped after withdrawal, if it is properly designed, and especially if the spermatozoa are found several times in succession, their probable location in the uterine mucus can be predicated. In some cases it will be found that actively motile spermatozoa have disappeared from the cervix after the lapse of a number of hours but are still found in the uterine mucus. In these cases the test is practically complete.

This study of the process of fertilization while it is actually in progress seems most rational and is in many cases extremely satisfactory, though care must always be used in its interpretation, as will be developed further later. The results obtained from it have led me to be a believer in the probable existence of that much mooted phenomenon, relative fertility; that is, I can now believe that a woman with slightly altered secretions may be sterile to a man with only moderately vitalized spermatozoa, and yet fertile to a man whose abundant and highly vital spermatozoa can resist her slightly hostile secretions; while, on the other hand, the moderately vital spermatozoa of the first man might succeed in effecting conjugation with the ovum through the absolutely normal secretions of another woman. On this latter point I have had fairly direct evidence, that is, I have seen instances in which with improvement in the secretions of the woman comparatively poor spermatozoa became able to make effective progress.

The Huhner test, valuable as it is, must however not be relied on too far lest it lead us into a too mechanical view of the problem of sterility. It requires for its successful use considerable tactile skill and no inconsiderable familiarity with the microscopic appearances to be noted, and there is undoubtedly much yet to be learned, from the microscopic point of view, by wider experience in the use of this test. It is not adapted for experimental, empiric use by the general practitioner, nor is it safe unless carried out with the most complete asepsis.

The several observations which may be made by this method will now be summarized, and their bearing on the results of other methods of examination will then be discussed.

If the vaginal pool when submitted to the microscope contains no spermatozoa, alive or dead, the probability is strong that the man is aspermatic and this should then be confirmed by direct examination of the semen as obtained by expression or from a condom specimen. Such aspermia may be merely temporary and is frequently neither permanent nor hopeless; but into the prognosis and treatment of aspermia and azoospermia I do not here propose to enter. If the vaginal pool contains an abundance of spermatozoa which are either dead, or at best feebly motile, at the time of a reasonably prompt examination, the character of the vaginal secretion is probably responsible for their death, and should in most cases be altered by treatment; but the importance of the vaginal condition is much affected by the size and position of the os uteri. There are not a few cases of widely opened os, with normal cervical secretions, in which a reasonable number of living spermatozoa succeed in entering the cervix in spite of a hostile vaginal secretion, that is, before it takes effect on them. If they succeed in entering the cervix in sufficient numbers and with sufficient vitality to be found later in the uterine mucus the condition of the vaginal secretion is of course of but little importance. If, however, as is frequently the case, spermatozoa are found, in an apparently normal cervical secretion, either dead or in a condition of limited vitality while the majority of their brethren have been killed by a hostile vaginal secretion, it becomes probable that even the most successful ones were largely devitalized by the latter, and its treatment is of the utmost importance.

Much the same thing may be said of the hostile conditions of the cervical secretion; but it may be remarked, in passing, that it is extremely interesting to see how often actively motile spermatozoa may be seen to progress across the field of the microscope in a cervical secretion of grossly normal appearance, until they come in contact with some clump of pus cells which is evidently tied together by sticky secretion, with which the tail of the spermatozoon becomes entangled. The result then is that he indulges in futile struggles to escape, by the violence of which he may be seen to become exhausted, and in a few minutes gives up the struggle and lies still. This is of course due to the admixture with normal serum of thick inspissated mucus from inflamed cervical glands. In these cases the cervical mucous membrane must of course be rendered normal before impregnation is likely to occur. It may here be again remarked that this is unlikely to be effected to the degree of normality which permits of impregnation, without an intelligent alteration of the size and shape of the os and cervical cavity by a plastic operation, in addition to a curettage and thorough if not repeated disinfections of the mucous membrane.

These conditions as actually seen under the microscope, then, amply demonstrate the reason for the almost invariable failure, in sterility cases, of the mere dilatation and curettage in which the general practitioner so often indulges, not infrequently, too, with results which permanently decrease his patient's chance of fertility under any treatment. At least such has been the result of my observations in this class of cases.

If the uterine mucus contains spermatozoa which have penetrated there and then died prematurely (they should live many hours if not days in this situation), it becomes probable that they have been killed by exposure to the tubal secretions so soon as they have reached the point where those secretions are but little if at all diluted by the secretion of the uterus, and those of the lower portions of the tract through which the spermatozoa have lived. If the uterine cavity contains fairly numerous spermatozoa of high and persistent vitality in a woman who nevertheless remains persistently sterile, the demonstration that her sterility is ovarian is sufficiently satisfactory to be practically useful.

By this means of direct observation of the progress of the spermatozoa through the genital canal, of their comparative vitality at the start and in each stage of their progress, an experienced observer may obtain information of the utmost value. In his interpretation of these facts, however, he must be guided not merely by these results, but by their correspondence with the observed local conditions both gross and microscopic, and by these as checked by his remembrance of all the light gained from the history, and from his study of the general condition of both partners. Otherwise I believe that he will take an unduly narrow view and will be in the long run none too successful in his management of these cases.

Success in diagnosis and prognosis from such complicated observations as these must always be a matter of the personal equation, but with sufficient care and thorough study they become increasingly accurate and often surprisingly so.

The prognosis in individual cases may now be discussed in accordance with the classifications by causations originally proposed.

If the male is azoospermatic the prognosis is that of azoospermatism, which varies with its cause.

If his spermatozoa are either few, abundant but somewhat lacking in motility, or in any other way imperfect, the prognosis which would be derived from the condition of the woman is impaired by just the amount of the feebleness of the male, and though it is usually not hopeless, both elements must be remembered in forming it.

If the spermatozoa are not only abundant but also long tailed, well formed, and active, the prognosis can be made from the condition of the wife alone.

When, in such cases, the only abnormality found is in the character of the vaginal secretion, or in such alteration in combination with a pinhole-sized and badly placed os, the prognosis of fertility under appropriate treatment is that of almost certain success. When, with first class spermatozoa, the abnormality is found in the cervix with an apparently normal uterine body, tubes and ovaries, the prognosis after appropriate treatment is always very good. When, with first-rate spermatozoa, the abnormality is apparently to be found in the uterine body, that is, when the uterine secretion as obtained by the syringe is sticky, or unduly filled with clumps of leukocytes; when the ordinary symptoms of endometritis are present; when the bimanual examination shows the uterus large and soft; but, on the other hand, when a careful bimanual examination under anesthesia satisfies the attendant that there is every probability that the ovaries and tubes are normal, the prognosis under treatment is good. When the abnormality is believed to be slight but existent in both tubes, that is, when both tubes are palpable though not greatly enlarged, the prognosis, though not necessarily hopeless, is not good. When both tubes are grossly diseased the prognosis is, in my opinion, so poor that operation is not justified for sterility alone unless both partners insist on it after full statement of the poor prognosis. When coincidence of all the above methods of examination leads the observer to believe that though one tube is undoubtedly or probably abnormal there is reason to believe that the other tube is normal, the prognosis is again good, after the removal of the affected tube. I have had several most satisfactory successes in such cases, though we must, of course, be always prepared in these cases to find that the second tube is occluded in spite of our belief to the contrary. When the whole genital canal is normal or substantially normal as shown by the result of an inspection and examination under anesthesia, with the support of the presence of active spermatozoa at the fundus, that is, when the fertility is demonstrably merely ovarian, when arrest of development is not present, but the ovaries are either normal or slightly enlarged, the prognosis after conservative operation on the ovaries is thoroughly good. In my opinion such an operation is justifiable under the conditions of today for sterility alone, provided that all the pros and cons have been placed before both parties and that both of them request operation after due consideration of them.

In the far more common cases in which there is an admixture of several of these abnormalities the prognosis must be determined for the individual case by carefully weighing the principles set forth above as applied to the individual combination of circumstances.

The results obtained in the treatment of sterility have long been, and too often are still, proverbially poor. I believe that the reason is to be found in the fact that so many physicians treat these cases from a purely empiric point of view and without any attempt at educating themselves in the special subject of sterility.

In the first place, the importance of an examination of both partners is too frequently overlooked; in the second place the search is too often directed to the discovery of lesions which should create ill health rather than toward the often minor conditions which determine sterility. To judge from my own experience, sterility is about as frequently the fault of the male as of the female, but popular opinion usually places the responsibility for the sterility on the woman, and this popular superstition is too often shared by the profession. I regret to say that my daily experience teaches me that many gynecologists do not hesitate to treat women and even subject them to operations, for sterility alone, with no knowledge whatsoever of the condition of their husbands. I feel bound to confess that in earlier days I have done it myself.

On the other hand, while urologists constantly rail at this weakness of the gynecologic portion of the profession, study of their writings inevitably leads one to the conclusion that too many of them have not plucked the beam from their own eyes. I have seen too many cases in which expert urologists have based their opinion on the sterility of a couple on an examination of the man alone to doubt that this branch of the profession is also often at fault. If the examination of a man shows him to be aspermatic no examination of the wife is necessary until his case has been concluded, but if, as so often happens, spermatozoa are present but are of doubtful excellence, the prognosis of the case must depend on the results of the examination of both partners. In this class of cases the examination of the spermatozoa as taken from the female genitals is of especial value, since it makes it possible to check at one sitting both the urologic and the gynecologic examinations, and to estimate their relative importance.

Nothing is more common than to have a woman referred from a distance unaccompanied by her husband, who is, however, stated by their attendant to be "all right"; and then to find that the statement that the husband is normal means merely that he is in general good health and potent, and does not mean that his spermatozoa have been seen. The treatment and more especially the operative treatment of a woman for sterility alone without actual inspection of her husband's spermatozoa is entirely unjustified. It is certainly practically expedient, and probably justifiable, to treat for sterility, even in an operative way, women who have been referred from a distance unaccompanied by their husbands, who present sufficient causes for sterility in their own person, and who bring an authoritative statement that the husband's spermatozoa have been examined and found normal, but the advantages to be gained by the inspection of the spermatozoa in their progress through the woman's genital tract, though not in my opinion essential, are nevertheless so considerable that sterility patients should, whenever possible, come to the specialist accompanied by their husbands.[3]

The case against the profession goes further than this common failure to study the couple as a pair, however. It may almost be said that the usual course of the gynecologist confronted by a case of sterility is to treat it from the standpoint of health and not from that of the relief of sterility, that is, to institute treatment or perform operations, directed to the removal of anatomic or other alterations which he perceives in a woman's genitals, without stopping to consider whether these observed peculiarities have anything to do with her individual sterility or not. It may almost be said that when the average gynecologist fails to detect any cause for sterility he dilates and curets the woman for the sake of doing something. There are of course many men whose conduct of such cases is conscientious and able, but the above description is, I believe, not too strong a statement of average facts, and has in my experience, in part at least, been applicable to the practice of some men who in other departments of gynecology are of recognized preeminence. Such empiric treatment is worse than useless. It too often renders futile, future rational efforts for the relief of the conditions which are actually important in the given case.

I believe it is mainly by reason of these two faults on the part of the profession that the treatment of sterility is so frequently unsuccessful. I believe that when sterilities are, as a habit, managed by the examamination of both partners as soon as sterility has become probable and before the woman has been subjected to useless and usually harmful minor treatment and operations, its prognosis will become what it ought to be and what it today is in well-managed cases, usually satisfactory.

321 Dartmouth Street.

---

3. A satisfactory examination of a couple for sterility cannot always be concluded in a single office visit. It may not infrequently require a number of visits, sometimes at intervals of several days.

ABSTRACT OF DISCUSSION

Dr. John O. Polak, Brooklyn: I wish to emphasize one point in connection with what Dr. Reynolds has said in regard to the fertility of the man. This point should be taken into consideration in every case; i. e., the male's past performances. I always have the man examined not only as to his potency, but as to the presence of evidences of previous infection, because that link—the history of previous infection—has a great influence on his potency.

Dr. Joseph B. DeLee, Chicago: My associate, Dr. Lespinasse, has been working on cases which I have referred to him, to see if we could not reach a solution of the difficulty presented by those cases in which the husband is well and the wife is well and yet sterility exists. He has worked in the light of the knowledge given us by recent studies in serology. We all know of certain instances in which the husband, after a divorce from the sterile wife, has secured children from another woman, and the wife, on remarriage, has also been fertile by another man. I, personally, have such a case under my present care, having delivered the woman twice after a second marriage, and a physician in Los Angeles having delivered the second wife of this woman's former husband.

Why did not the spermatozoa of the first husband succeed in fertilizing the ovum of the first wife? Lespinasse has found the secretions in different women dissolved the spermatozoa of different men—a sort of immunity reaction. Experiments are being made, but I am not yet able to give the results, since we want to accumulate a sufficiently large number.

When Dr. Reynolds mentioned the change in the local secretions, this is but a step further in the study of the gross symptomatology and pathology of the genital tract. We have got far enough in the study of these immunity reactions that it seems possible we may find the cause of sterility where the husband presents no evidence of disease, has strong, living spermatozoa, and where the wife has no pelvic inflammation or no real surgical pathology of the parts.

The treatment of sterility has been, in a manner, extremely routine, and therefore, unsatisfactory, and women are bandied about from one specialist to another until they lose faith in medical art.

Another point that will explain some of the causes of sterility is the abnormality of the internal secretions. I hesitate to make that statement because it throws us into an immense field that is very dimly lighted by positive knowledge, but I do know cases that have been unsuccessfully treated elsewhere and have been successfully treated by the glands of internal secretion—thyroid and other extracts. In some instances administration of these preparations has been followed by impregnation, especially that type of firm fat obesity, in which the women are round and plump and the fat is hard, almost like firm flesh, and the periods are inclined to be irregular and small in amount. Those cases have responded to combined treatment occasionally.

The use of alkaline douches just before intercourse deserves mention. The husband, as a cause of the sterility, must be always emphasized, and I have found that excessive smoking of tobacco is occasionally a cause of sterility, and that alcohol, even when the spermatozoa are alive and motile, indirectly prevents them from successfully fertilizing an ovum; that workers in arsenic, antimony, and other chemicals, in spite of live spermatozoa are sometimes sterile. Then I have had men who have had syphilis and are sterile, even though the examination of the semen showed motile spermatozoa. The sperm injected into the woman has both a local and a general effect. It has been demonstrated that the spermatozoa not used for fertilization enter the cells of the genital tract and are absorbed into the cell. This is a line of light on the immunal theory. Isn't it possible that a woman can be immunized; her serum so protected against the advent of the spermatozoa that it dissolves them when they come? Perhaps this explains—when the husband or wife has been sent away for six or eight months—successful fertilization. The law of incompatibles thus bids fair to be explained.

Dr. H. O. Pantzer, Indianapolis: His, the anatomist, said that the complexity of the genitalia in the human female is such as to make it, to him, a surprise that woman ever conceives. Regarding the nervous excitability referred to, I have this observation to mention, that women who have delayed menstruation frequently give evidence of a presenile sclerosis of the ovum. These cases are often associated with chronic intestinal auto-intoxication. This interrelation of toxemia and ovarian sclerosis is not surprising when we recall that toxemia strikes essentially at all glandular organs, and in all is followed by withering and sclerotic changes. It is surprising how many cases of spanomenorrhea or amenorrhea are helped by looking after systemic elimination. All will remember the reliance the older practitioners and gynecologists placed on elimination, as evidenced by the free laxative remedies invariably contained in their prescriptions.

Dr. Edward Reynolds, Boston: Some of the points about which Dr. DeLee spoke were omitted in my reading, but were in the paper.

I do not think the bicarbonate of soda routine for the acid vagina is a good thing. The acid nature of the vaginal secretions is, in all probability, merely the most superficial indication of the chemical changes which destroy the spermatozoa. The failure of such treatment in the vast majority of cases is because we only neutralize the acidity and not the other chemical alterations. I am unable to speak as yet of various studies which I have made, and have had made, and am making on the chemical and microscopic character of the secretions. So far as I know, the chemical and microscopic examination of the mixed secretion of the male and the female, as obtained from the female genitals, is, as yet, an entirely virgin field. There have been a number of men who have observed the spermatozoa and their action in those fluids, but the essential point which we cannot yet speak of is the microscopic and chemical examination of the mixed secretions; the establishing of a normal standard and the detection of abnormality. I have learned to recognize certain arrangements of pus cells, and have seen the spermatozoa swimming freely, come into one of those pus cells, tangle his poor little tail in it, stop his progress, thrash, thrash, thrash, and lie dead. You have to reduce that apparently normal cervical secretion. There are dozens of such things that we know nothing of. The question of immunity is a very curious and interesting one but from a practical standpoint on both the question of abnormal chemistry and immunity we must be careful how we determine our action in such cases by subjects that are so little worked out that our knowledge is hardly a gleam in the obscurity of our ignorance.

THE ACTION OF RADIUM ON CANCERS OF THE PELVIC ORGANS

A CLINICAL AND HISTOLOGIC STUDY

HENRY SCHMITZ, M.D.

CHICAGO

Since April, 1914, I have treated 112 cases of malignant growths of various regions of the body with radium. Forty-eight of these occurred in pelvic organs. Forty-one of these pelvic cancers are considered in this paper. Thirty-six were in the uterus, five in the rectum and three in the bladder. The tumors were inoperable, recurrent or operable carcinomas. Twenty-four were inoperable, nine recurrent and eight operable.

Ten of the inoperable and three of the recurrent carcinomas were thoroughly cauterized or excochleated and then cauterized preceding the application of radium. Broken-down tissue and débris were thereby as completely removed as possible, and the extent of the intensity of the gamma rays into the depths of the tissues correspondingly increased. The operable cases were subjected to an extensive vaginal cauterization and an abdominal panhysterectomy. As soon as the patient recovered from the operation, radium was inserted into the crater of the broad ligament. The rays were used as a prophylactic to recurrence.

I wish to draw attention to the remarkable deodorizing and purifying action of radium. Those who have attended patients after such abdominal panhysterectomies well remember the sloughing of tissues in the crater of the broad ligament, which gives rise to a terrific putrid odor and discharge and an irregular temperature. One, or at the most two applications of radium stop these distressing complications. The cauterizations always were performed with ordinary soldering irons at red heat.

THE TECHNIC

The technic of applying the radium varied as to the limiting of time of the applications and the kind of metal filters used, but not in the amount of milligrams of radium element applied (uniformly 50 mg.).

In the beginning of my radium work, the duration of each application was from ten to twelve hours, occasionally twenty-four hours. The interval between the treatments varied from seventy-two to ninety-six hours. These applications were continued until a decided improvement occurred in the subjective as well as the objective condition of the patient. This usually took place after a dosage of from 3,000 to 4,000 milligram hours had been reached. The treatments were then given weekly and finally biweekly, until the condition of the patient warranted a cessation of the treatments. Frequent examinations were insisted on to keep the patient under control. A total dosage of from 8,000 to 10,000 or more milligram hours was thus recorded.

Fourteen patients were treated in this manner (Cases 2, 5, 6, 7, 8, 9, 10, 11, 12, 13, 15, 16, 17, 18). A subjective improvement was usually noticed after the third application. The pain decreased, the profuse purulent, creamy discharge became scanty and serous, and the hemorrhage ceased. The general state of health improved correspondingly. After about 3,000 milligram hours of radium element had been given (that is, after from about twenty-one to twenty-four days, the bimanual findings became usually normal. In a few cases such a state was not reached until about 6,000 milligram hours had been applied. The uteri which were firmly fixed at the first examination became freely movable and could be plainly outlined. The adnexa were palpable and the crater in the cervix

TABLE 1.—CANCERS OF PELVIC ORGANS TREATED WITH RADIUM

Case No.	Name of Patients	Hospital Number	Date of Adm.	Uterine	Rectal	Milligram Hours Radium Element	Operable	Recurrent	Inoperable Cauterized	Inoperable Not Cauterized	Remarks
1	Mrs. B.	Augustana 41218	9/24/14	+		4,200	+			+	Cauterization 11/3/14.
2	Mrs. H.	Augustana 40098	5/22/14	+		9,685		+			Op. four years ago.
3	Mrs. H.	Augustana 40717	7/23/14	+		10,850				+	
4	Mrs. D.	Augustana 40044	8/25/14	+		6,775	+				
5	Mrs. E.	Augustana 39516	8/23/14		+	9,900		+			
6	Mr. J.	Augustana 40405	6/29/14		+	3,150			+		
7	Mrs. K.	St. Mary's 25176	6/30/14			2,175	+	+			Cauterization 9/16/13.
8	Mrs. K.	Augustana 24058	8/13/14			5,700	+		+		
9	Mrs. McQu.	Augustana 39778	4/23/14			6,520			+		
10	Mrs. McO.	Augustana 39516	8/23/14	+		3,375			++		Became operable.
11	Mrs. M.	St. Mary's 24098	8/17/14	+		7,500				++	Became operable. Carc. corp. uteri.
12	Mrs. P.	St. Mary's 23967	3/7/14	+		7,875					Became operable.
13	Mrs. B.	Augustana 40270	6/11/14	+	+	2,675		+	+		Also cauterization.
14	Mrs. C. S.	Augustana 40082	6/4/14	+		9,280					Became operable.
15	Mrs. Th.	Willard Hosp.	4/4/14	+	+	8,513		+	+	+	
16	Mrs. V.	Augustana 39631	8/4/14	+		9,048				+	
17	Mrs. W.	Augustana 39755	4/19/14	+		8,585				+	
18	Mrs. W.	Augustana 39469	3/19/14	+		8,700			+	+	
19	Mrs. P.	Augustana 40508	7/14/14	+		8,760					
20	Mrs. J.	Augustana 40456	7/4/14	+		3,500					
21	Mrs. R.	Augustana 40649	6/22/14	+		1,125			++		
22	Mrs. Sk.	Augustana 41305	10/7/14	+		4,000			+		
23	Mrs. B.	Augustana 41321	9/25/14	+		6,900				+	
24	Miss Bo.	Washington Bvd. 9098	10/17/14	+		4,150					Carc. corp. uteri.
25	Mrs. H.	Washington Bvd. 9092	10/1/14	+		8,675		+		++	
26	Mrs. M.	West Side 23965	11/21/14	+		2,300				++	Cauterized 11/23/14.
27	Mr. St.	St. Mary's 29967	11/27/14	+		4,150					Sarcomatous myoma?
28	Mrs. St.	Augustana 41944	12/29/14			3,000			+		
29	Mrs. T.	St. Mary's 27006	1/5/15			3,500					
30	Mr. To.	Augustana	1/23/15			2,400			+		
31	Mr. A. M.	Willard	2/10/15			4,500					
32	Mrs. M.	Augustana 42319	2/15/15			5,175					
33	Mrs. H.	Post-Graduate	2/6/15			4,900				+	Colored.

was covered with healthy granulations, being protected by a grayish or whitish membrane. The parametriums also were free of any indurating bands. In other words, by cautious procedures and careful observation, we established the fact that on an average from 3,000 to 4,000 milligram hours of radium element were necessary to attain an apparently objective cure.

This knowledge led to the second mode of treatment, which I may term the "intensive method." Just as maximum dosage of Roentgen rays may be concentrated into the possibly shortest space of time, so the milligrammage of radium element might be given within the shortest limit of time, and from 3,000 to 4,000 milligram hours of radium element were applied within from sixty to eighty consecutive hours.

Ten cases in particular (Cases 1, 3, 4, 14, 20, 23, 25, 26, 27 and 28) were thus treated. Although we obtained the same primary results as with the first method, we, however, noted the following points:

1. The apparently objective cure was not reached any sooner than with the first method.

2. The associated symptoms were exceedingly stormy and much severer. They consisted, chiefly, in a marked loss of weight, strength and appetite, with hyperpyrexia, obstinate vomiting, profuse diarrheal stools and obstinate dysuria. Although these symptoms were only transitory, lasting from eight to ten days, the patient suffered much, a condition which we rarely observed in the cases treated by the first or "intermittent method." If such manifestations did occur in this method, they were very mild and of very short duration, lasting usually a day or two.

3. Destruction, ulceration or necrosis of the tissues was of regular occurrence. Repair of these defects was slow. Fistula formation, vesicovaginal, rectovaginal or even intestinovaginal, occurred in ten cases. However, I wish to state that fistula formation existing at the time of the beginning or taking place during the first few days of the course of the treatment must

TABLE 2.—INOPERABLE CANCERS TREATED WITH CAUTERIZATION AND RADIUM

Case Number	Cause of Inoperability	Date of Cauterization	Total Mg. Hrs. of Radium Element Applied	Primary Results — Duration of Treatment	Further Treatment	Results and Present Condition
9	Involvement of bladder and parametrium	4/23/14	6,320	5/12/14 to 7/ 5/14	None..........	Died from bladder and vulva invasion.
11	Involvement of bladder and rectum	3/18/14	1,750 3,200 2,550	4/14/14 to 4/23/14 6/17/14 to 7/23/14 8/12/14 to 8/23/14	.... None.	re- marks sult return
12	Extensive involvement of parametrium and rectum	3/ 8/14	7,875	4/ 2/14 to 6/11/14	July 14, 1914. Abdominal panhysterectomy	Died Dec. 20, 1914 from invasion of rectum.
16	Involvement of parametrium	3/ 5/14	9,043	4/ 1/14 to 9/ 9/14	April 24, 1914. Abdominal panhysterectomy	Well. Pelvis normal.
18	Marked cachexia...	3/20/14	8,700	4/ 1/14 to 7/31/14	....	Died August, 1914 from invasion of bladder and exhaustion.
22	Extensive involvement of vaginal vault	10/ 8/14	4,000	10/17/14 to 10/22/14	....	Died December, 1914 from exhaustion.
23	Extensive involvement of vagina and parametrium	9/25/14	6,800 1,200	10/19/14 to 11/ 1/14 2/ 9/15 to 2/11/15	....	Well. Pelvis normal.
29	Involvement of anterior vaginal wall	1/ 6/15	8,500	1/21/14 to 1/24/15	Repair of vesico-vaginal fistula March, 1915	Well except fistula.
39	Involvement of parametrium	3/16/15	8,700 350	3/20/15 to 4/ 4/15 4/25/15	....	....
40	Involvement of bladder and parametrium	4/ 7/15	5,050	4/15/15 to 5/ 6/15	....	June 11, 1915; metastasis of right inguinal glands. Panhysterectomy
36	Pyometra; involve-	3/10/15	2,925	3/12/15 to 3/23/15	....	

be ascribed to the extensive cauterization. The damaging action of the radium rays is a contributing cause (Cases 1, 4, 6, 15, 20, 26, 29 and 46). While fistula formation occurring from three to four weeks after the beginning of the radium applications must be directly attributable to the destructive action of radium, and extensive invasion of the bladder or bowel with cancer forms the predisposing cause (Cases 2, 8 and 33).

Finally, the following plan of treatment was adopted and carried out in the rest of the cases: A course consists of from six to eight séances of from ten to twelve hours each, with an interval of from thirty-six to sixty hours. This course is followed by an intermission of three weeks. If a bimanual examination made at this time reveals an apparent cure, two or three applications of from 500 to 600 milligram hours of radium element are given every second or third day. Another interval of three weeks is allowed, and if the examination then reveals a normal condition, the treatment is considered terminated. Negative findings, of course, are followed by another course of from 3,000 to 4,000 milligram hours. This "interval method" gave the best subjective and objective results with a minimum of concomitant symptoms, so that I consider it the method of choice.

Lead filters of 1, 2 and 3 mm. thickness were used in my first work. A 1 mm. filter was deemed sufficient for intra-uterine applications, while the heavier filters were employed in vaginal, rectal and vesical cases. Following the advice of Adler, Werner and others, I soon replaced the lead with brass filters of from 1 to 1.5 mm. thickness. Whether or not the lead filters cause severer latent destructions of tissue than brass filters I am unable to prove. Such disturbances occurred either in very advanced cases of carcinoma, with breaking down uterine or vaginal walls, or in extensively cauterized tumors, as mentioned before. The secondary rays produced in the metal filters were

Case Number	Cause of Inoperability	Total Mg. Hrs. of Radium Element Applied	Duration of Treatment	Primary Results			Further Treatment	Result and Present Condition
				Refractory	Subjective Improvement	Objective Improvement		
2	Extensive involvement of vagina	9,525	5/30/14 to 9/24/14	....	Yes	....	....	Cauterization Nov. 3, 1913. Has vesicovaginal fistula; cachectic.
5	Involvement of entire vagina, rectum, vulva	9,900	6/1/14 to 8/19/14	Yes	....	....	....	Had colostomy. Died from exhaustion.
14	Involvement of right ureter and sigmoid	9,250	6/7/14 to 8/5/14	....	Yes	Yes	....	Aug. 5, 1914, abd. panhysterectomy; resection of sigmoid. Died Nov. 20, 1914, from carcinomatosis.
15	Involvement of parametrium and rectum	8,512	4/4/14 to 6/17/14	....	Yes	....	....	Oct. 10, 1913, colostomy. Died Jan., 1915; cancer of liver.
19	Chronic endocarditis with decompensation	8,750	7/19/14 to 8/9/14	Yes	....	....	....	Died, August, 1914, from endocarditis
21	Extensive involvement of rectum	1,125	7/29/14 to 8/8/14	Yes	....	....	....	Patient refused further treatment on account of rectal tenesmus caused by radium; had colostomy; died.
25	Cachexia and local extension of tumor	8,875	11/6/14 to 12/5/14	Yes	....	....	....	Died.
27	Pyosalpinx and involvement of abdominal organs	4,150	11/27/14 to 12/3/14	Yes	....	....	....	Died.
28	Extensive involvement of bladder	3,600	12/31/14 to 1/25/15	....	Yes	Yes	Dec. 31, 1914, cystotomy for insertion of radium	Died January, 1915, from exhaustion after hip amputation for path. fracture of femur due to metastasis.
30	Extensive involvement of bladder	2,400	1/31/14 to 2/2/15	....	Yes	Yes	Jan. 26, 1915, exploratory cystotomy	Bladder free from tumor mass; gained in weight and strength.
33	Cachexia; vagina and bladder invaded	4,800	2/6/15 to 2/22/15	Yes	....	Yes	....	Developed vesicovaginal fistula; refused to continue treatment. Died.
36	Pyometra	2,925	8/12-23/15 to 3/23/15	....	Yes	Yes	....	Cervix now normal.
37	Involvement of bladder	1,700	8/15/14 to 3/20/15	Yes	....	....	March 8, 1915, exploratory laparotomy	Had a thrombophlebitis. Exacerbation. Died from septicæmia.
31	Extensive involvement of rectum	4,800	2/12 to 4/2	....	Yes	Yes	....	Rectum normal and freely movable. Returned to work.

arrested by surrounding the filter with a cot made of pure Para rubber of a thickness of from 1 to 3 mm. The healthy vaginal walls were protected by snugly packing the vaginal canal with gauze, Para rubber or lead plates surrounded by rubber and gauze.

CLINICAL   RESULTS

Tables 2 to 5 show at a glance the results of the radium treatment. The amount of the milligram hours of radium element used, and beginning and duration of the treatment and the present condition are enumerated for each case. Of the ten cases of Table 2, one case was refractory, and nine cases evidenced a subjective and objective improvement. Objective improvement indicates negative findings on bimanual palpation. Five of this group have succumbed to the disease. One has remained well since April, 1914, one since October, 1914, and one since January, 1915. Two cases, 39 and 40, are of too recent date to permit an expression as to the remote results. The primary results, however, are very good. Three of these cases (12, 16 and 18) were subsequently subjected to an abdominal panhysterectomy.

Fourteen inoperable cases, enumerated in Table 3, were treated only with radium. They were far advanced or extremely cachectic cases or had constitutional manifestations contra-indicating even a cauterization. Ten have died or are slowly succumbing to the disease. Four are free of all objective and subjective symptoms. They, and three cases not yet listed, were treated only recently; and considering the poor results obtained in the other ten cases, I must withhold a final opinion. One case (Case 14) had, after the completion of the radium treatment, a panhysterectomy.

Of the nine recurrent carcinomas, listed in Table 4, five show an entirely refractory behavior toward the radium rays. Four revealed a subjective and three also an objective improvement. One of the latter

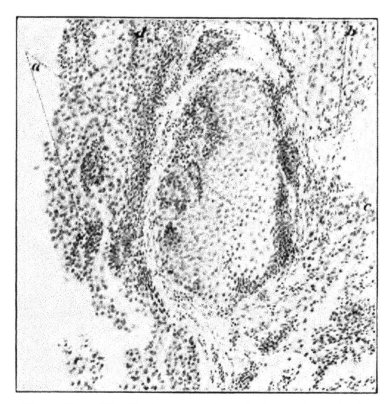

Fig. 1 (Case 33).—Carcinoma, portio vaginalis, cervix uteri. Low power reproduction of tissue removed Feb. 6, 1915, at beginning of treatment: *a*, squamous cell carcinoma; *b*, connective tissue; *c*, lymphocytic infiltration; *d*, area reproduced in Figure 2.

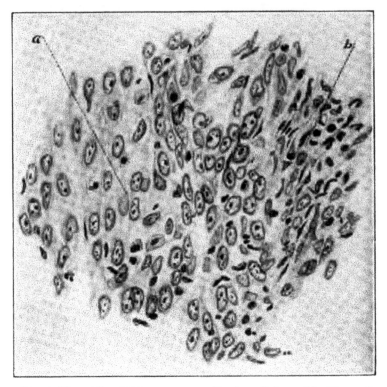

Fig. 2 (Case 33).—High power magnification of Area *d* in Figure 1:
a, carcinoma cells; *b*, connective tissue.

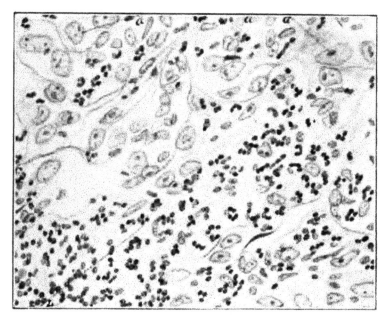

Fig. 3 (Case 33).—High power magnification of tissue removed Feb. 18, 1915, after 2,400 milligram hours of radium element had been applied from Feb. 6 to 8, 1915: *a*, enlarged carcinoma cells; *b*, lymphocytic infiltration; *c*, note connective tissue fibers surrounding groups of carcinoma cells.

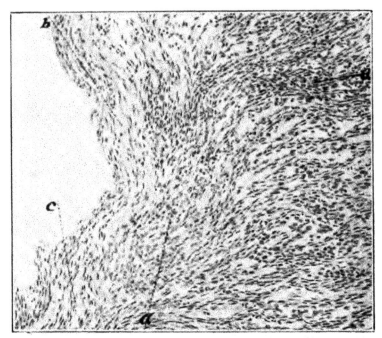

Fig. 4 (Case 33).—Low power magnification of a section of tissue removed Feb. 28, 1915, after 4,800 milligram hours of radium element had been applied from Feb. 6 to 8 and Feb. 18 to 20, 1915: *a*, carcinoma cells; *b*, connective tissue cells; *c*, area reproduced in Figure 5 under high power.

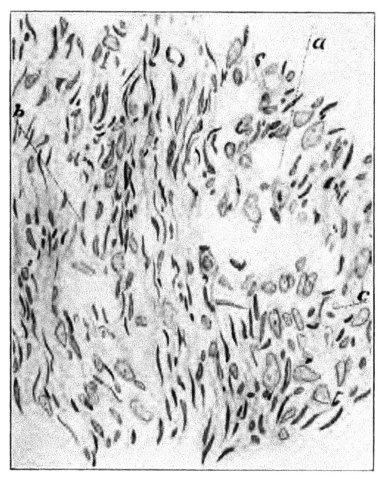

Fig. 5 (Case 33).—High power magnification of area marked *c* in Figure 4: *a*, area of necrobiotic tissue; *b*, area of connective tissue; *c*, cytolytic carcinoma cell.

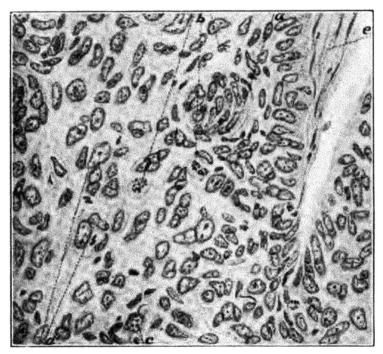

Fig. 6 (Case 39).—High power reproduction of cervical tissue removed March 16, 1915: *a*, nest of carcinoma cells; *b*, karyolysis of nuclei; *c*, granulation of protoplasm; *d*, vacuolation of protoplasm; *e*, connective tissue.

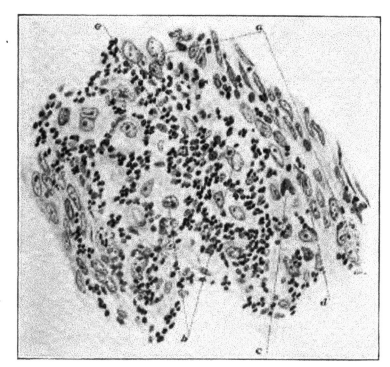

Fig. 7 (Case 39).—High power magnification of tissue removed from center of cervix, March 28, 1915, after 1,600 milligram hours of radium element had been applied from March 20 to 26, 1915: *a*, degeneration of nuclei; *b*, granulation of protoplasm; *c*, degenerating carcinoma cell; *d*, mitosis of cell; *e*, lymphocytes.

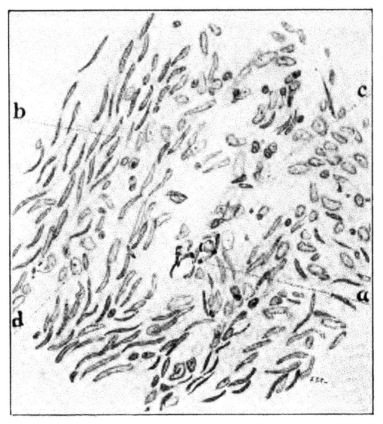

Fig. 8 (Case 39).—High power magnification of tissue removed April 7, 1915, after 3,700 milligram hours of radium element had been applied from March 20 to April 4, 1914: *a*, macrophagia-connective tissue cells; *b*, connective tissue cells; *c*, necrobiotic carcinoma cell; *d*, vacuolation of protoplasm.

Case Number	Character of Operation	Date of Recurrence	Condition of Pelvic Organs	Duration of Treatment	Primary Results		Remarks and Results
					Refractory	Objective Improvement	
8	Vaginal panhysterectomy	June, 1914	Nodule and ulcer size of bean in vaginal vault	7/27/14 to 11/30/14		Yes	Patient succumbed to an intercurrent disease, March, 1915; cauterization 7/31/14.
8	Abd. hysterectomy. Vag. cauterization	Sept. 1913	Involvement of entire vagina	4/ 6/14 to 5/28/14		....	Vesicovaginal fistula. Died Sept. 21, 1914, from exhaustion.
10	Vag. hysterectomy	Oct. 1913	Involvement of vagina, vulva and perineum	4/25/14 to 5/18/14			Septicemia after third radium treatment. Died May, 1914.
18	Vag. hysterectomy	Apr. 1914	Involvement of entire vagina	6/13/14 to 6/15/14			Vagina healed immediately; did not return for treatment.
20	Vag. hysterectomy, salpingo-oophorectomy sinistra	Mar. 1914	Mass involving right adnexa	7/10/14 to 7/18/14			Developed vesicovaginal intestinovaginal fistula; succumbed to exhaustion August, 1914.
26	Abd. panhysterectomy	Nov. 1914	Ulcer in vaginal vault	11/28/14 to 11/25/14			Nov. 23, 1914, cauterization of vag. vault; developed intestinal fistula; died Dec. 27, 1914; exhaustion.
32	Vaginal hysterectomy	Apr. 1914	Ulcer in vaginal vault involving right parametrium and bladder	2/15/15 to 3/28/15			April 20, 1915, tumor increasing in size; patient loses weight and strength; has much pain.
34	Abd. panhysterectomy	....	Mass involving vag. vault extending to right up to brim	8/ 9/15 to 8/20/15			Losing weight and strength.
35	Vag. and abd. panhysterectomy	Aug. 1914	Ulcer involving entire vagina and right parametrium	3/10/15 to 4/ 6/15			April 30, 1915, vagina and vulva normal and free of any nodular masses.
45	Percy cautery. Abd. hysterectomy	Never compl. recovery	Crater involving parametril	6/ 1/15 to 6/12/15			

patients died eight months after the beginning of the
treatment from an intercurrent disease. She had had
a recurrence the size of a pea, which disappeared after
radium treatment and cauterization. Another patient
after a successful primary result did not return for
a reexamination, and has not been heard from. The
third one has again a healthy vagina, and the pelvis is
free from indurating masses, though the entire vaginal
canal was a mass of carcinomatous growths extending
up into the base of the right broad ligament and down
into the fourchet.

Of the eight operable cases (Table 5) treated by
surgery and radium, one patient died nine months
afterward from a metastasis of the liver, another one
two months later from a severe hemorrhage from the
vagina. The others are at this time in a normal condition and do not show a recurrence. The average
time elapsed since the operation is eight months.

HISTOLOGIC FINDINGS

The action of the gamma rays on carcinoma tissue
has been studied in eight cases, namely, six uterine
(Cases 12, 14, 16, 24, 29 and 39) ; one rectal (Case 31),
ane one skin cancer (Case 85). The latter has been
added, as it affords a particularly favorable instance
for the study of the changes occurring in carcinoma
cells by the action of radium. The reproductions of
the first microscopic sections (Figs. 1 and 6) were
made from tissues removed from the tumor before
the beginning of the radium treatment. The time of
removal of the other sections is stated beneath each
illustration; also the amount of radium element applied
preceding the removal of the sections, and the time
duration of the application of each course.

The histologic changes may be divided into four
stages :

The first stage is characterized by an enlargement
of the carcinoma cells, a hyperchromatosis and a pyk-
nosis of the nuclei. They are evident in all the cases

TABLE 5.—CANCERS TREATED BY SURGERY AND RADIUM

Case Number	Date of Operation	Character of Operation	Complications of Convalescence	Mg. Hrs. of Radium Element Applied	Duration of Radium Treatment	Result	Remarks and Present Condition
1	9/25/14	Abd. panhysterectomy; vag. cauterization	Vesico abd. and vesicovag. fistula	4,400	10/10/14 to 10/26/14	Perfect recovery	Died two months afterward from a vaginal hemorrhage.
4	8/26/14	Vag. cauterization; abd. panhysterectomy	Vesicovaginal fistula	6,775	9/ 5/14 to 10/13/14	Recovery, but fistula	Well, April, 1915; fistula closed.
6	7/17/14	Perineal cystotomy and cauterization	None	8,150	8/ 8/14 to 9/ 1 14	Recovered.	
7	7/ 2/14	Resection of 9" of rectum; perineal operation	None	2,175	7/16/14 to 8/ 1/14 and 10/30-31/14	Recovered.	Dying from metastatic cancer of liver.
17	4/20-24/14	Vag. cauterization; abd. panhysterectomy	None	3,525	5/15/14 to 5/20/14	Recovered.	
24	10/29/14	Abd. panhysterectomy	None	4,150	10/21-23 and 11/11-13/14	Recovered.	Oct. 21, 1914, diagnostic curettage; well.
38	3/16/15	Abrasion of mucosa; amputation of cervix	None	2,550	3/21 to 3/28/15	Recovered.	
41	4/16/15	Vag. cauterization; abd. panhysterectomy	None	3,960	4/19 to 5/4		Extensive involvement of anterior vaginal wall. Really an inoperable case; impossible to remove entire growth.
44	5/20/15	Abd. panhysterectomy; cauterization	None	4,000	5/23-31/15		Extensive involvement of right parametrium; impossible to remove entire tumor mass.

examined.   These changes usually occur within about
ten days after the first application of radium (Figs.
3 and 7).

In the second stage we observe karyolysis, karyor-
rhexis, cytolysis and cell detritus.   Figure 3 shows
many evidences of such changes.   They are observed
as early as from the first to the third week of the
treatment.

The third stage shows an absorption of the cellular
and nuclear débris by phagocytes.   Macrophages and
microphages are concerned in this step.   Microphagic
activity is highly evident in Figure 3, while macrophages are seen to be active in Figure 8.

The fourth stage is the stage of connective tissue
proliferation and scar formation.   It completes the
histologic cure of cancer.   The places left vacant by
the dead carcinoma cells are immediately filled by
young fibroblasts derived from the connective tissue
stroma of the tumor.   The fibroblasts become differentiated.   Figure 4 shows the connective tissue regeneration.   The fourth stage appears usually after from
the first to the third month, but may occur much
sooner.

A difference frequently exists between the clinical
results and the histologic findings.   For instance, in
Case 12 there was evidence of a completely destroyed
cancer tumor, yet the patient succumbed to a bowel
invasion, proving that some cancer cells either
remained uninfluenced by the radium or regenerated
after the subsidence of the action of the rays.   Therefore, certain questions arise which call for definite
answers before we can positively state that radium rays
cause a degeneration and ultimate death of cancer
tissue and a simultaneous regeneration of connective
tissue.

1. Are we able by histologic examination to differentiate the necrobiotic changes in the carcinoma cells
brought about by natural and artificial conditions from

those caused by the influence of radium rays? It is evident that we cannot do so. Cells undergo necrobiotic changes in the course of their existence. Heat, caustics and alcohol, brought in contact with the tissues, may produce the same changes, as is well known. However, such general and extensive changes as seen in these specimens, the absence of cell degeneration as evidenced in the first sections, and, finally, the regularity of their occurrence in all the tissues investigated, even in those not previously cauterized, permit us to state that they must be caused by the action of the gamma rays.

2. Can we, by examination of small pieces of tissue removed from the growth, determine the extent and intensity of the action of radium rays? We cannot from such an examination, but could do so from serial sections of all the organs removed either intra vitam during operations, or, preferably, postmortem.

I have, fortunately, four cases in which an abdominal panhysterectomy was performed after a clinical cure of the cancer by the use of radium rays was obtained (Cases 12, 14, 16 and 24). Serial sections were made from the tissues removed. A microscopic examination revealed that the cytolytic changes were generally present throughout the organs removed. This does not prove that distantly located foci were not left behind. As a matter of fact, Patients 12 and 14 died subsequently from cancer. This shows that viable cancer cells were left behind somewhere in the pelvis. Bumm examined tissues acted on by gamma rays and removed afterward during postmortem examinations. He estimated that the intensity of the gamma rays sufficient to destroy carcinoma tissue extended into a radius of 4 cm. Within this area of intensity, carcinoma cells were not found present; beyond it, however, typical unchanged cancer cell nests were still found to exist. In other words, extensive carcinoma growths are only partially destroyed by gamma rays. This area of destruction, however, has a diameter of 8 cm., and enables us to reach tissues which a knife could never remove.

3. Is it possible by such microscopic examinations to state whether a carcinoma cell has perished or whether it might not regenerate after the action of the radium rays ceases? The following citation will illustrate the answer to this question: Chéron and Rubens-Duval treated a patient suffering from an inoperable carcinoma of the cervix with radium during November, 1910, and January, 1911. The patient was apparently clinically cured. She died from an intercurrent disease (a cerebral softening) during April, 1912, fifteen months after the beginning of the radium treatment. All the internal organs and tissues were removed postmortem, and a careful serial histologic examination of all the tissues did not reveal a single carcinoma cell at any place of the organism. A complete anatomic cure by radium rays has thus been demonstrated.

My investigations demonstrate the uniformity and general extent of the necrobiotic changes brought about in the carcinoma cells by the action of the gamma rays. Bumm's researches fix the extent of the area of intensity of the rays within which a carcinoma will become destroyed, and Chéron and Rubens-Duval's case proves the capability or efficiency of the radium rays to bring about an anatomic cure of cancer.

CONCLUSIONS

1. The best method of applying radium is the interval method by which from 3,000 to 4,000 milligram hours of radium element are applied within from about fourteen to twenty-one days.

2. The alpha and beta rays must be arrested by a brass filter of from 1 to 1.5 mm. thickness.

3. The secondary rays, forming in the metal filter, are rendered inert by a rubber cot of from 1 to 3 mm. thickness.

4. Inoperable cancers that are not far advanced so that cauterization is not contra-indicated yield satisfactorily to radium therapy.

5. Advanced inoperable and recurrent cancers are ordinarily refractory toward the radium rays. Any improvement is at least very temporary.

6. The patients treated with the rays after surgical removal of the organs have done well, although the time elapsed since the treatment averages eight months.

7. Patients suffering from cancer should be treated surgically and then radiologically, and if surgery is contra-indicated they should receive radium treatment, which at least relieves the subjective symptoms and often the objective ones.

8. The time elapsed since the commencement of the radium treatment in all the cases enumerated is too short to permit definite opinion as to the remote results of radium treatment.

9. Clinical and histologic studies enable us to pronounce the radium rays a valuable addition to the therapy of cancer.

10. It will require years of constant observation to demonstrate such results as anatomic cures.

11. The same measure that is applied to establish the efficacy of surgical procedures in cancer treatment must certainly be employed in radiotherapy.

Finally, I wish to thank my colleagues at the Augustana, St. Mary's and Willard hospitals, and especially Dr. A. J. Ochsner, for the encouragement they have given me to carry on these investigations by referring clinical material. Without their assistance it would have been impossible to record these extensive clinical observations.

25 East Washington Street.

RADIUM IN THE TREATMENT OF CAR-
CINOMAS OF THE CERVIX UTERI
AND VAGINA

———

HOWARD A. KELLY, M.D.
AND
CURTIS *F.* BURNAM, M.D.
BALTIMORE

———

The scope of this paper has been intentionally limited to a consideration of the value of radium in treating the malignant epithelial new growths of the vagina
and cervix uteri. Equally interesting technical problems and clinical phenomena are met when radium is
used in treating other kinds of malignant tumors, for
example, the sarcomas and carcinomas, and tumors in
other organs, as the bladder, breast, tongue, etc. The
technic, the indications for treatment and results
obtained vary with the type of tumor and its location
so greatly that each demands separate consideration.
It is especially difficult to have to exclude the adenocarcinoma of the fundus uteri, as it is quite radiosen-
sitive and as we have of it the most excellent material,
both clinical and anatomic. The problems connected
with its surgical as well as radium treatment, however,
differ widely from those of the cervical—uterine and
vaginal — cancers.

Absolute valuation of a therapeutic agent is obtainable only after all methods of using it have been tried
out on carefully selected and classified cases over a
period of years. Our knowledge of the curative action
of radium on cancers of the uterine cervix and vagina
is as yet in its infancy; nevertheless, its ultimate possibilities, viewed in the light of present experience,
seem very great. That it does greatly increase the per-

centage of the curable cases of these cancers and correspondingly diminishes the percentage of the incurable is already evident and demonstrable.

So far as is known, untreated cancers of the cervix uteri and vagina do not heal spontaneously and do inevitably lead to painful death after a period of suffering varying from a few months to several years.

The continuous and painstaking work and investigations of many surgeons and pathologists through a period of more than two decades have firmly established the accepted surgical technics with their proved five-year cures. During this time there has been accumulated an immense store of information regarding the occurrence, the etiologic importance of trauma, the histopathology, the avenues of extension, the rate of growth and the complications of these malignant, epithelial new growths.

The Wertheim radical hysterectomy, in our opinion, yields a higher percentage of permanent cure in cancer of the uterine cervix than does any other operative procedure. It affords, however, much less help in the treatment of primary cancer of the vagina.

Nothing is more misleading than a gross statistical statement of so many patients operated on, such a primary mortality and so many permanent cures. The operator who takes only the early and moderately advanced cases has a lower primary mortality and a higher permanent cure rate than does the one who treats many of the border-line operable type. Where a professional and public educational campaign against the disease has been carried out, as in Vienna, the proportion of easily operable cases is much larger than where such advanced methods have not been followed. Great need exists for reports on carefully classified groups of cases, and not only the extent of the growth but also its histologic type should be taken into account in the group separations.

A statistical report by Howard A. Kelly and J. Craig Neel of the cases of uterine cervix cancer seen at the Johns Hopkins Hospital up to August, 1913, shows 57 per cent. operable, 11 per cent. primary mortality and 25 per cent. permanent cure. It is of interest that only one case of adenocarcinoma remained free from recurrence for two years after the operation. Wertheim[1] states that 50 per cent. of his cases are operable, and that 50 per cent. of those patients operated on remain well. Krönig[2] states that not more than 20 per cent. of the cervix cancers are permanently cured by operation and less than 5 per cent. of the primary vaginal cancers.

The present report is based on a series of 213 cases' of cancer of the uterine cervix and vagina treated with radium at the Howard A. Kelly Hospital, between Jan. 1, 1909, and Jan. 1, 1915. Although one of the cures dates from 1909, it was not until December, 1912, that we secured sufficient radium and developed sufficient enthusiasm to employ it systematically, and indeed only in the last eighteen months have the patients in the operable class been invariably radiated as well as operated on. Of the 213 cases, fourteen were operable and 199 inoperable or inoperable recurrent cancers. We have refused treatment to no inoperable case that has come to the hospital, although we have discouraged the coming of patients with evident general carcinomatosis. Before passing to a detailed analysis of these cases and the results obtained by treatment, it seems necessary to discuss very briefly some questions of technic, of histologic change (in radiated tissue) and of theory as to the mechanism of the action of the rays on tissues both, normal and pathologic.

It would be most profitable here to digress into a most fascinating field of human knowledge, but time does not permit even a bare outlining of the physical properties of radium. Suffice it to say that radium is obtainable in stable form as a bromid, chlorid or sul-

1. Wertheim: Strahlentherap., iii, 537.
2. Krönig: Strahlentherap., iii, 28.

phate, and that by appropriate means radium emanation, a gas, can be separated from the radium salts.

In order to carry out such a radium radiation, as the cases under consideration require, it is necessary to have applicators which hold either dry radium salts or the emanation of radium. The emanation has a great advantage in that it is possible to vary the size, shape and strength of the applicator at will and for each case; it requires, however, considerable skill in glass blowing and in mercury vacuum-pump manipulation.

Figure 1 shows a few applicators; the millimeter rule permits an easy estimation of size. The small tube between the needles is a glass capillary in which any amount of emanation between a fraction of a millicurie and a curie (equal to a gram of radium) can be placed. This can be inclosed in a metal container of its own shape and length, or it may be placed in the outer end of one of the record syringe hypodermic needles, shown on either side of it. Immediately to the right of the needle is an applicator containing 100 mg. of pure radium chlorid in a glass tube encased in a thin platinum envelope 0.4 mm. thick, and all covered by a small rubber cot about 3 m.m. thick. Still further to the right is shown the platinum envelope necessary to hold 100 mg. of pure radium chlorid. The last figure to the right shows a small flat applicator. These can readily be made an inch or two in diameter, and will hold immense or small amounts of emanation as desired. Through the glass container are emitted from the radium two kinds of rays: the beta and the gamma.

The beta ray is particulate matter, a negatively charged ion, deflectable by an electromagnet, entirely absorbed by 3 mm. of lead, or 2 cm. of tissue. Occurring in ten times the quantity of the gamma rays, it produces much more marked destructive biologic effects.

The gamma ray is a vibration of ether of extremely short wave length. It is comparable to ordinary light and the Roentgen ray. It is extremely penetrating, passing through inches of lead or feet of tissue.

When tested by the heavy metals, such as lead, platinum, etc., both the beta and the gamma rays vary as to penetration. There are soft, medium and hard rays of each class; however, according to Keetman and Mayer, the absorption of these rays in tissue is as if they were uniform, that is, for a given thickness of tissue there is an equal percentage of absorption of the rays going through it. The work of Keetman and Mayer carried out with mesothorium is being repeated with radium in our physical laboratory, but is not yet finished. According to them, 8 per cent. of the beta rays are absorbed by each one-tenth millimeter of tissue and 5 per cent. of the gamma rays by each centimeter of tissue. Beta and gamma rays can be used together or the gamma ray can be used alone by placing a 2 cm. lead screen or a 1 mm. platinum screen between the radium and the part treated.

In addition to absorption in tissue, another most important factor in determining the intensity of radiation, on any surface, from a uniform source, is the distance from the source; for the intensity as in all spherical dispersion varies inversely with the square of the distance. If, for example, we place 1 mg. of radium 1 mm. distant from a 1 mm. square surface and then extend the distance to an inch or 25 mm., the intensity at 1 mm. distance is 625 times that at the distance of 1 inch, as can be readily calculated.

Taking the 1 mg. at 1 mm. in one second on 1 square mm. of surface, as the unit of dosage, and taking in the factors of spherical dispersion and tissue absorption, the following table shows the effects at various depths and the quantity of radium necessary to produce a unit dose in one second when the applicator is placed 5 cm. away from the surface.

A factor not considered in the table but of the highest importance, is that, within certain limits, increasing the duration of the application correspondingly diminishes the amount of radium required to produce the unit energy: for example, a unit dose at a depth of 5 cm. can be secured with 1 gm. radium in 12.88 seconds, or with 200 mg. of radium in a little more than a minute.

Thickness of Tissue Traversed, cm.	Absorption of Tissue, per Cent.	Radiation Transmitted, per Cent.	Dispersion Correction	Intensity of Radiation per sq. mm.	Amount of Radium Unit to Give One mg.
0	0	100	0	1	2,500
1	5	95	0.695	0.66	3,788
2	9.75	90.25	0.51	0.464	5,410
3	14.3	85.7	0.39	0.335	7,465
4	18.6	81.4	0.31	0.251	9,960
5	22.17	77.83	0.25	0.194	12,880
6	26.06	73.94	0.207	0.153	16,310
7	29.76	70.24	0.174	0.122	20,480
8	33.3	66.7	0.147	0.098	25,500
9	36.7	63.3	0.128	0.081	30,850
10	40	60	0.11	0.066	37,500

Figure 2 shows graphically the changes in intensity of gamma radiation at different depths in the tissue.

It is evident that when beta radiation is needed in the depths, it can be secured by placing the emanation-containing needles at equal distances, never greater than 1 cm. from each other, throughout the entire area to be radiated. When gamma radiation alone is used, it should be borne in mind that the greater the distance the radium is placed from the surface, the greater the relative penetration secured in the depths. The ideal radiation is a homogeneous and equal one throughout the entire affected volume.

Consideration of the above facts makes it clear why to do extensive work adequate amounts of radium are necessary, and why the statements of so many milligram hours with such and such filters mean little or nothing unless the distance worked at is clearly stated. It is also, we think, evident that each case must be individualized and appropriate radiation given. In cancers along the vaginal wall, especially on the rectal side, it is of advantage to have flat applicators and to get within a few millimeters of the vaginal surface, as in this way the infected vagina gets a maximum and the rectum a minimum radiation. In radiating the regional lymphatic glands or upper parametrium, a number of portals should be used from the abdomen, back, vagina and perineum, at distances varying from 2 to 5 inches from the surface. Figures 3 and 4 show schematically the common locations and distances of the cervical and vaginal cancers from the body surface. We propose in a separate communication to deal exhaustively with the technic of radiation and will not go into further detail here.

Excellent descriptions of the histopathologic changes found in the cancerous uterine cervix after intense radium radiation can be found in the reports of Hansemann[3] and Haendly.[4]

Beginning a week after radiation there is swelling of the cell protoplasm, hyperchromatosis and pykenosis of the nuclei. After five or six weeks, the cancer cells are entirely gone, the connective tissue and blood vessels show hyalin changes. There may be a marked infiltration with polymorphonuclear leukocytes, and often giant cells are present. At a later stage this necrotic and inflammatory tissue is replaced by ordinary connective tissue. When radium is placed directly within the cervix and left sufficiently long, changes of this type invariably occur.

We have eight uteri removed a sufficient time after radiation to study the changes in the tissues. Vestiges of cancer have been demonstrated in only three of these. All will be serially sectioned and reported on in detail in a later communication. All were from patients with cancers originally inoperable.

It should be borne in mind that the intense inflammatory changes described above follow overradiation

3. Hansemann: Berl. klin. Wchnschr., 1914, No. 23, p. 1064.
4. Haendly: Berl. klin. Wchnschr., 1914, No. 2, p. 86.

and are due to imperfect technic. The action of the rays is not in a true sense specific; normal tissues as well as pathologic are injured and can be easily destroyed. There are wide variations in the resistance to radiation in different normal tissues. The vaginal wall and cervix are very resistant, enormously more so than skin. Bumm of Berlin gave currency to a widely accepted dictum that the limit of the gamma-ray efficiency (in tissue) was 4 cm. It is probably true that it is not possible to place radium directly in the cervix and radiate sufficiently to destroy the cancer cells beyond 4 cm. without causing severe local destruction of normal tissues; but it is possible to radiate from almost any distance by proper disposal of the applicators. In one case we cleared up an extensive vaginal cancer by radiation through the vulva, the radium being placed 10 cm. from the surface of the vulva. In another patient who did not recover, but died of general cancer, we saw large metastatic deposits disappear from the iliac lymphatic glands—the patient was thin and the masses easily outlined.

Our view of the action of radium is that, to markedly varying degrees, it injures all tissues, and that the injury is some kind of intracellular chemical change. It seems to us improbable, however, that the disappearance of cancer cells without any demonstrable effect on normal cells can be due solely to a difference in resistance of the cells to radiation. The common observation that in two cases with the same type of growth, subjected to the same radiation, different results are obtained; that in one the cancer disappears promptly and in the other is not affected at all, suggests the importance of resistance in the patient. It also opens up a wide field for speculation and experimental investigation as to what this resistance may be, where it is located, how it may be artificially produced, etc.

Radiation carried to the extent of severe injury of normal tissue may defeat its own ends. We have observed in one specimen of uterine cancer and several specimens from other parts of the body a condition which needs interpretation. In the cervix cancer the facts are as follows: The patient came in with solidly fixed parametria; intense intracervical radiation was given with the result that the uterus became freely movable; after six weeks hysterectomy was performed. Microscopic study showed from within outward, (1) a zone of necrosis; (2) a zone of greatly modified connective tissue, blood vessels and altered cancer cells; (3) a zone of normal connective tissue and no cancer cells.

In every patient treated, a radiation up to but not beyond this toleration of the normal tissues should be given so as to take in all the infected area, including the parametria and regional lymphatic territory. This radiation should be made as homogeneous as possible, bearing in mind the underlying physical principles already mentioned.

The most easily injured normal tissue in connection with cervical and vaginal cancer radiation is the rectum. In our earlier cases, when we were less familiar with our agent and totally unacquainted with the tissue reactions, this complication was not uncommon and in some cases led to such serious results as ulceration, fistula formation and even death from infection. Such a complication manifests itself first in from ten days to two weeks after the application, by diarrhea and tenesmus. In the mild types this may disappear in two weeks and no further trouble develop. In the severer grades the proctitis lasts two months or more, then disappears to recur about the beginning of the sixth or seventh month, with ulceration in the anterior rectal wall. This condition is very painful and takes from three to five months to heal. In the worst cases actual fistula formation takes place before healing. *We are*

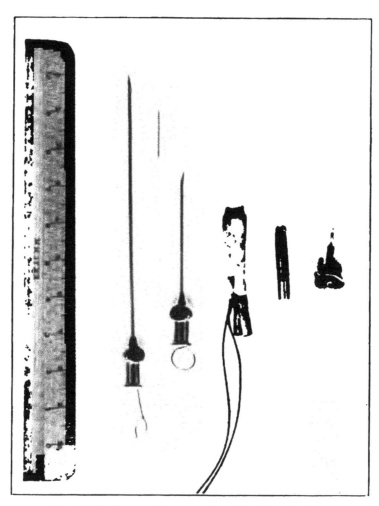

Fig. 1.—Radium applicators and scale indicating size.

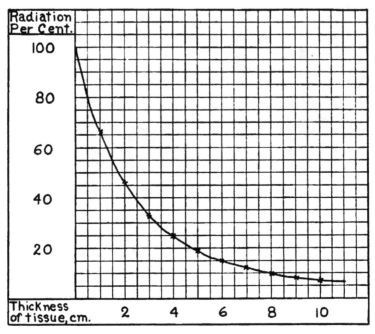

Fig. 2.—Curve showing the variation of the intensity of gamma radiation with the thickness of tissue.

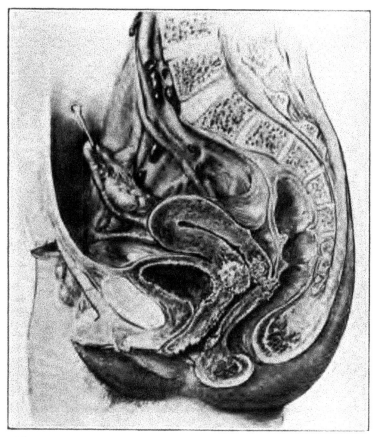

Fig. 3.—Common locations and distances of the cervical and vaginal cancers from the body surface as seen from the side.

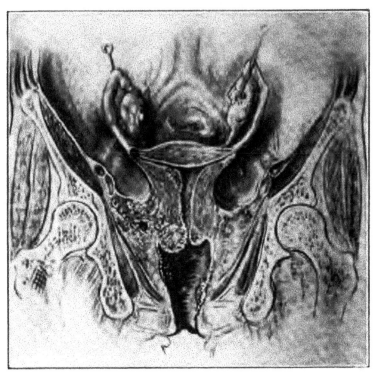

Fig. 4.—Common locations and distances of the cervical and vaginal cancers from the body surface as seen from the front.

happy to state that this complication can be avoided in every case. We have not seen it for months.

The first radiation should be given in a single dose, following which a pause of at least five or six weeks is necessary before a second treatment is given. During this time the patient should be examined once a week. Some carcinomas, especially the basal celled of the vaginal wall, begin diminishing in a few days and disappear in as short a period as two weeks after the treatment. Most of them begin the decrease at the end of two weeks and continue diminishing for five or six weeks. If at the end of six weeks the growth has disappeared, another four weeks should pass before a second treatment is given. After the second treatment practically all cases in which there will be recovery will show complete disappearance of the growth. In view of the fact that we have seen a number of recurrences developing several months after apparent complete disappearance of the growth, we believe that the radiation should be repeated every few months for a year or two. Some of our permanent successes have been, however, secured from a single radiation.

As a rule, the general symptoms which follow a radiation are mild nausea for twenty-four hours and a sense of weakness for four or five days. Sometimes there are no disagreeable symptoms at all, and in no case has there been any alarming developments. The patients are rarely kept in the hospital longer than the day of treatment.

Every patient before treatment is most thoroughly investigated both from the local and general standpoints, and invariably tissue is secured for microscopic study. The application of the radium sometimes made under nitrous oxid is more frequently made without anesthesia.

Up to the present time we have not found means of determining prior to radiation what its effect will be. The general strength of the patient is not of prime importance. We have seen local disappearances in

patients in the last stages of general carcinomatosis.
Nor is the extent of local involvement of importance;
large growths may disappear and small ones fail to do
so. The histologic type is likewise relatively unimportant in this connection; in the cured list are twenty-
nine squamous-celled epitheliomas, seventeen basal-
celled epitheliomas and seven adenocarcinomas. In
passing, we desire to state that squamous-celled epitheliomas may long remain local, and that some basal-
celled epitheliomas rapidly metastasize. Among the
recurrent cases, it has been noted that those which
develop late, two years or more after operation, almost
always do well; the cause most likely is connected with
immunity factors in the patient.

CLASSIFICATION AND DEFINITION

We have divided our cases into three groups:
1, operable; 2, inoperable; 3, recurrent inoperable.
The results obtained have also been placed in three
classes: 1a, clinically cured; 2a, improved; 3a,
unimproved.

1. By operable cancers are meant those still confined to the cervix or only moderately involving the
parametria and vaginal walls. They are not fixed to
the pelvic wall on either side and have not caused
hydronephrosis and are not associated with pelvic pain.

2. By inoperable cancers are meant those associated with general metastasis, those firmly fixed to
one or both pelvic walls; those extensively involving
the bladder, vagina or rectum. In short, cases in which
we have never cured the patients by operation.

3. By recurrent inoperable cancers are meant such
recurrences following operation as we have never
cured except by radium.

1a. By clinically cured is meant the complete disappearance of the cancer so far as palpation, curettage
or other method may disclose associated with the
apparent perfect general health of the patient.

2*a*. By improved is meant a definite betterment of the patient's condition. In the lesser degrees this may consist of a cessation of hemorrhage and discharge, or a disappearance of pain which has resisted all the drugs, including morphin. Among these, too, are placed twelve cases in which all local trouble disappeared, but the patient showed metastasis at the time of treatment or developed it subsequently. Two of these patients were found locally free of cancer at necropsy, and in two, in whom hysterectomy was carried out after apparent clinical cure, the uteri are clear of the disease, in spite of the fact that both patients are now dead from general metastasis. In most of the cases of this group the reduction in the size of the tumor was marked. It also includes some early cases in which the treatment was very imperfect.

3*a*. By unimproved is meant no material benefit having been produced. Most of these showed histologic improvement on microscopic examination of curettings. In more than two thirds of them the disease was immense and the general condition of patients bad.

All of the patients included in this report were treated prior to January, 1915, and the cured ones were apparently cured at that time. All of the cured have been investigated by one or both of us personally, with a few exceptions in which the examinations were made by competent men. The last report on each case was obtained in May, 1915.

RESULTS

The results obtained by the treatments may be summarized as follows:

Out of the 213 cases treated, 14 were operable and 199 inoperable.

Operable Cases.—Of the 14 operable cases, 10 patients were operated on and treated prophylactically with radium. Of these, 2 have been well for more than three years, 1 for more than two years, 4 for more than a year, and 3 for more than six months. The number is too small to draw conclusions from, and yet is suggestive, when we consider that in 75 per cent. of all cases with operation there is recurrence and that 60 per cent. of these recurrences take place within one year following the operation.

In four cases of the operable group, on account of some general contraindication to operation, radium alone was used. All of this group are living and well; 2 for over three years and 2 for over one year.

Inoperable Cases.—The total number of inoperable and inoperable recurrent cases is 199, of which 53 patients have been clinically cured, 109 markedly improved and 37 not improved.

Our series includes 35 cases of originally inoperable cancer of the cervix uteri or vagina in which the patients are clinically cured; in 2 cases for over four years; in 2 cases for over three years; in 4 cases for over two years; in 17 cases for over one year; in 10 cases for over six months. It also includes 18 cases of originally inoperable recurrent cancers in which the patients are now clinically cured; in 1 case for over six years; in 1 case for over four years; in 11 cases for over two years; in 10 cases for over one year; in 5 cases for over six months.

Excluding the operable cases, in which we have both operated and used radium, there are 203 cases left; in 57 of these 203 cases the patients are clinically cured. We employ the word clinically cured and will reserve the word cured for later reports, to apply to cases beyond the five-year limit, which has been conventionally adopted by surgeons as a time limit for estimating the permanency of cures of malignant disease.

Of the 57 clinical cures, 1 has lasted for six years; 3 for over four years; 4 for over three years; 5 for over two years; 29 for over one year, and 15 for over six months.

CONCLUSIONS

We are convinced that radium is of exceedingly great value in the treatment of cancers of the cervix uteri and vagina.

We expect with all confidence that the results in the next 200 cases will far surpass those reported here.

We again emphasize that the betterment in the improved but not cured cases is so marked that it alone makes radium a great addition to existing methods and would justify its use.

We believe that every inoperable cancer of the cervix uteri or vagina, provided general metastasis is not evident, stands a chance of at least 1 in 4 of cure by radium treatment.

There is a marked reason to believe not only that a large number of inoperable cases are curable, but that by the joint use of radium and operation that the 1 in 4 cure rate of operation in operable cases may be raised to 3 in 4 or better.

We have seen that some cervical cancers do not respond to radium treatment. This same variation in reaction occurs in many other types of neoplasm. It is apparently due to a lack in the patient of resistance to the specific growth. Work should be directed toward determining where the body products which attack a radiated cancer arise and what they are. On account of the certainty that some of the operable cancers of the cervix would not be cured by radium and also on account of the necessity of having many patients over five years cured in order to be sure of the permanency of the results, we advise, in operable cases, hysterectomy and radiation. This is the rule in clearly operable conditions. In border-line cases, we advise the use of radium, as the permanent cures from operation are not numerous in this group. If the growth does disappear, it can only be determined whether or not hysterectomy is advisable by trying out both methods; this as yet has not been done in a

sufficient number of cases to arrive at any definite conclusions. We do feel, however, that when clinical
cures have occurred in inoperable cases, operations are
probably best not carried out. Manifestly an inoperable case which becomes operable but does not entirely
heal should be treated by operation.

Finally we desire to restate most emphatically that
radium can and should be used in these cases without
any local or general injury to the patient treated.

1418 Eutaw Place.

ABSTRACT OF DISCUSSION

ON PAPERS OF DRS. SCHMITZ AND BURNAM AND KELLY

Dr. J. F. Percy, Galesburg, Ill.: Ewing of New York said
a few years ago that the balance in cancer is easily upset;
and this must be true, because there are a number of methods of destroying or inhibiting cancer that have a certain
number of clinical cures to their credit. It would be
interesting if we could go back in a historical way to these
various methods and determine just how much they have
accomplished. One thing has been brought out by both
of these papers, and that is the totally inexplicable way
some cases are clinically cured and other cases apparently
of the same type are either made worse or not affected by
the same treatment. The problem of the treatment of inoperable cancer of the uterus has always been of the gross
mass, and it is a question whether or not radium, in the
great mass of cancer usually seen in the cervix, is as valuable
as some other method that will at once, or in a comparatively
few minutes, get rid of this gross mass. Another problem is the metastasis, and I am glad that both the essayists
have mentioned an immunity, or, at least, suggested it. This
immunity is undoubtedly developed in greater or less degree,
and without doubt takes care, in many cases, of the metastases after the destruction of the gross mass. At least
I am convinced of this from my own experience. I am especially interested in the destruction of the gross mass by
heat. I am convinced that this method is the most certain of any of the methods that have been brought to our
attention. In addition, it does not require specialized judgment and the apparatus required is comparatively inexpen-
sive. One of the difficulties of radium and the Roentgen
ray in attacking the gross mass of cancer, is that they
break down a lot of cancer cells, and if drainage is not provided, an overdose of the broken-down cancer cells may
be absorbed and kill the patient. In other words, even

with radium or the Roentgen ray, if one attacks the gross mass he must provide for some form of drainage. This is easily done with the heat technic. It is not easily done with either radium or the Roentgen ray.

DR. S. M. D. CLARK, New Orleans: The two papers show definitely that we are not marking time in the warfare on cancer. We are beginning to see rays of light, and I feel confident that if the present pressure is kept up, our results will progressively improve. I am sorry that I cannot discuss the subject from the radium point of view, but since I note that the best results obtained by one of the essayists was when using the radical operation after the growth had been transformed by using radium, it seems appropriate to consider cancer of the uterus from another angle.

Though the Percy heat method has great merit, still when viewed in the light of a cure, it falls short and is to be looked on more as an adjunct or link in the chain of treatment. Time is too short to go into the detail of my combination method, but its chief point rests in being able to transform inoperable into operable cases by performing the work as a two-stage operation. At the first sitting the abdomen is opened and both internal iliacs and one ovarian artery are tied, primarily for the purpose of starving the growth, as well as to control secondary hemorrhage. Heat is applied at the same time. After three to five weeks' interval the patient is transformed constitutionally and locally, when the radical removal is done. This method increases operability and decreases the primary mortality. If we keep accurate records of our work, in ten years stock can be taken of our results and then the best method can be adopted.

DR. HENRY SCHMITZ, Chicago: It is a question of developing first the therapy, and second the technic of the application of radium. If we do know the amount and the manner in which we should use it, our results will improve. My first cases treated were not so successful as at present. I feel that radium will do more in the eradication of cancer than any other means. I have applied surgery, heat and everything I possibly could use, but since I have been using radium I feel more confident of benefiting my patients.

DR. CURTIS F. BURNAM, Baltimore: I omitted one thing that I intended to say, that in the beginning we catheterized and curetted our big masses. More recently we are not doing that. So far as I know, there is no general upset in the treatment. We give a single treatment, repeat it in six weeks if the growth is still there. If it has gone, we wait three months; but if it has not gone we repeat; and the patient rarely stays in the hospital longer than the day of treatment.

SUBINFECTION FROM FOCI IN THE PELVIS AND ABDOMEN

HORACE G. WETHERILL, M.D.
DENVER

Much detailed study, both clinical and bacteriologic, has resulted in establishing many important facts relating to general infections of mouth and tonsil origin, while little, very little, appears to have been given to like pathologic processes of pelvic and abdominal origin.

Perhaps an exception may be made of acute general infections, such as follow mechanically induced abortions, gonorrhea, etc., though there is still much to be learned about their bacteriology and routes of diffusion; the phenomena of arrest in the lymph nodes and in certain organs like the liver and spleen, and the vital processes by which such infections are combated and immunity is established.

Chronic infections from local foci in the pelvis and abdomen, or as Adami prefers to call them, subinfections (and toxemias caused by toxic products liberated by the death of the organism), have failed to receive the attention their importance merits.

Sir Arbuthnot Lane has drawn the attention of the medical world to what he calls autointoxication of intestinal origin, and he aims to cure the condition through a total extirpation of the colon. His work and conclusions, however, appear to have been based in the main on clinical data with what, in this generation of laboratory requirements, would seem to be insufficient checking with systematic bacteriologic investigations of the primary source of the disease or of the carriers of the "toxin"; the blood and lymph and the vessels and organs through which they pass.

Lane's reasoning and results have, therefore, failed to convince many surgeons that the hazardous operations he advocates are justifiable for the relief of the various, often trivial, and far too numerous diseases and symptoms he cites as curable by short circuiting and colectomy and, happily, humanity has been spared the indiscriminate adoption of a practice which would inevitably be disastrous if generally accepted and applied.

Of this Adami says, "It is, I hold, too grave a responsibility to assume, this of starting an epidemic of operative surgery purely upon an empirical basis, on a foundation that is not established upon uncontrovertible fact."

The acceptance of Lane's theories as to the causes of many of the diseases he attributes to colonic stasis implies the acceptance of the theory of the permeability of the normal colon by pathogenic organisms; a theory which would appear to have been clearly disproved by Neisser, who asserts that "the importance of the intestine as a portal of entrance for bacteria has been greatly exaggerated." He further says, "It has been shown that under certain *pathologic conditions* some bacteria may enter the blood stream through the intestinal wall as, for instance, anthrax, tubercle bacilli, typhoid bacilli and some of the colon group. Some authors have assumed that such a passage of bacteria through the intestinal wall may take place under normal conditions or when there are only slight changes, such as venous congestion. Attempts have been made to explain many diseases whose etiology was not clear in this way." Neisser reviews the literature and gives a bibliography of seventy-five titles. He describes experiments of his own, which show that under normal conditions bacteria do not pass through the intestinal wall either into the blood or lymph circulation. In contrast with Nocard's results, he found that after bacteria were given to animals, both the chyle and the mesenteric glands were completely sterile. He found also that the chyle has no bactericidal qualities.

As gynecologic and abdominal surgeons we are more often and more directly interested in the invasion and diffusion of pathogenic bacteria through damaged tissues such as may be found following more or less acute inflammatory processes involving the fallopian tubes, the appendix, the stomach and duodenum, and the gallbladder. During the process of recovery such infections are accompanied by partial immunization on the part of the patient, a reduced virulence on the part of the pathogenic organism and by an effort on the part of the surrounding tissues to isolate, encapsulate or encyst the local focus of the disease.

This encapsulation, if ultimately accomplished, is brought about through a quarantine fibrosis by the adjacent tissues, but before this quarantine fibrosis is complete, and indeed to some extent afterward, there are leaks, and many organisms escape into the circulation, and there is in consequence a more or less prolonged period during which such pathogenic bacteria are taken up by the blood and lymph vessels and are carried to other portions of the body to form new foci by metastasis or to create new lesions in the tissues about certain terminal vessels, as in the heart, kidneys, brain, gallbladder, stomach and duodenum.

In the light of what is now known of general systemic infections from foci in the mouth and tonsils, every gynecologist and abdominal surgeon of wide experience can look back over his past work and recall a vast number of instances in which he has been able to cure such chronic, or subinfections, by the removal of some old focus in the pelvis or abdomen. The removal of old tubo-ovarian abscesses, a "chronic appendix," a thickened, contracted or strawberry gallbladder, has been followed by a restoration of general health and well being. With the analogy of the infections from the mouth and tonsils an open book before us it seems quite clear where and how the illness of our patients may have originated. We must not, however, be content with inferences and deductions from comparisons. We must know and we must know with the certainty that can come only through the bacteriologic study of specimens removed at operation, and of the blood and the lymph glands of such patients. The bacteriologist must work with the surgeon and the surgeon must work with the bacteriologist to solve these problems.

Billings enumerates the common systemic results of focal infection as follows:

1. Chronic arthritis as one of the most common.
2. Nephritis, both acute and chronic.
3. Cardiovascular degenerations.
4. Chronic neuritis and myalgia.

He cites among other local foci of infection, chronic ulcers of the gastro-intestinal tract, chronic appendicitis, cholecystitis and cholangeitis, and the genito-urinary tract. He says of chronic catarrhal appendicitis that it may produce not only the local discomforts, including disturbance of the functions of the digestive organs, but it may also be a focal source of systemic infection with the damage done chiefly to the cardio-vascular apparatus.

It was such a case as the preceding paragraph refers to that recently attracted my attention anew to this subject and inspired this paper. I venture to give a brief history of the case.

The young man had long been a patient of Dr. S. G. Bonney. Dr. Bonney had seen him through several severe attacks of diffused systemic infection of primary tonsillar origin with severe local manifestations in the heart, pleura, kidneys and appendix. A detailed history as to his early cardiac complications may be found fully set forth in Bonney's "Pulmonary Tuberculosis and Its Complications," pages 499, 500, 501.

The transcript of the history of this case as given to me by Dr. Bonney for this paper is as follows:

A tonsillectomy was recommended for a delicate child of 8 years with a history of repeated attacks of acute tonsillitis. The operation was done while visiting in another state, but on return to Colorado it was found that the tonsillar tissue had been but partially removed. The operation was in no sense a success, for subsequent acute attacks took place. When 10 years of age the first serious systemic complication was experienced.

During the ensuing few years he experienced several acute illnesses characterized by fever, pain in the joints, dilatation of the heart with endocardial murmurs and rapid pulse, these attacks occasionally being preceded by a mild tonsillar infection. Three years ago it was decided to have the tonsils thoroughly enucleated under a general anesthetic, notwithstanding the fact that the heart at that time was not in an entirely satisfactory condition, the pulse being rapid even when at rest and the heart murmurs persisting. There was also a slight nephritic involvement as evidenced by a trace of albumin with hyaline and granular casts. He was kept in bed for several months after the operation, following which the albumin disappeared, as well as the casts, and the evidences of kidney irritation have never returned.

In April, 1912, he went to Kentucky and Tennessee, remaining one year and two months, apparently in a very satisfactory condition, but in March, 1913, again experienced an acute illness reported to have been characterized by acute pains in several of the joints suggesting what had been previously regarded as acute articular rheumatism (undoubtedly an acute infectious arthritis). He remained in bed from March until June in the South, developing in the meantime an acute pleurisy with effusion *and a very severe appendicitis which was regarded as inoperable on account of his heart trouble.*

He was brought home in June, 1913, apparently hopelessly ill. There was great prostration and emaciation with daily fever of 101 to 102, marked dyspnea, dilatation of the heart and a double mitral murmur. He remained in bed for many months, I should judge at least six, the chief features of treatment being absolute and complete rest, and efforts to promote elimination in every possible way, together with supporting measures, careful attention to diet and stimulation.

He made a very satisfactory improvement and was finally able to be about without noticeable shortness of breath until an acute attack of appendicitis developed in the summer of 1914. Immediate operation was performed by Dr. Wetherill and the subsequent course has been satisfactory beyond measure. He has never had an ill day since. There has taken place a very substantial gain in weight, the pulse is uniformly slow and of good character, the color of the face is better than for ten years, there is no shortness of breath even on considerable exercise, there is no dilatation of the heart. There still exists a faint but distinct endocardial murmur with satisfactory compensation of the cardiac insufficiency.

My operation for the removal of his appendix was done July 26, 1914. The patient was then 18 years old. The attack was so severe that immediate operation was deemed imperative notwithstanding the bad condition of the heart. Every preparation was made for rapid work and the anesthetic was carefully given. The appendix was found gangrenous and covered with lymph. It was enveloped in a mass of old adhesions made up of the omentum and other adjacent tissues. Following my practice in such cases, no intraperitoneal drainage was used, but an ample drain was placed through the superficial tissues down to the peritoneum. The patient made an exceptionally smooth operative recovery and, as stated by Dr. Bonney, had been in excellent health since. Taking the history of the case and the findings at the operation together, it is probable that this old focus about the appendix was responsible for maintaining the systemic intoxication and infection.

Such an endocarditis as was present in this instance, originating through systemic infection from a focus which provided constant though minute doses of pathogenic organisms, and which is at once improved after the removal of the source of the infection, leads one to speculate whether most of such remote lesions are not truly embolic in origin.

If possible it must be determined also whether in such a case as this, for example, the infection of the appendix was primary in the appendix or whether it was due to, or coincident with the early attacks of tonsillitis for which the tonsils were removed and to which the early cardiac symptoms were attributed, or whether the infection of the appendix was secondary and possibly embolic from the tonsil focus.

It now seems highly probable that the transfer of many pathologic processes from one part of the body to another, which we have called metastases, are in truth a conveyance of the causal agent—the pathogenic bacteria—through the blood vessels, with their arrest in clumps or as individual organisms in the terminal vessels and the tissues surrounding them, constituting infective capillary emboli such as are found in pyemia and so-called ulcerative endocarditis from the *Streptococcus viridans*.

In confirmation of this theory Rosenow has demonstrated that the reason why acute rheumatic endocarditis originated only in youth is purely anatomical. The typical verrucose endocarditis of acute rheumatism is, he claims, of embolic origin and can be induced by inoculating half grown rabbits with streptococci of a grade of virulence closely allied to that which in older rabbits will induce myositis. Why the older rabbits do not suffer from endocarditis is because the heart valves have become nonvascular, the fine arterioles present in early life in the proximal two thirds of the cusps undergoing obliteration.[1]

In all probability similar vascular changes explain the incidence and location of rheumatoid changes at different life periods.

The application of such facts as are here set forth to the common types of neglected sources of infection in the pelvis and abdomen, must of necessity awaken all of us to a fuller realization of the possibilities of such local foci as causes of some of the subtle and intractable constitutional conditions presented by many of our patients.

The practical result of such application will be that no investigation of one of these cases of chronic systemic infection can be regarded as complete till all possible sources of focal infection have been investigated, which will include with the mouth and tonsils all other lymphoid masses, such as the appendix; and in adults, the genito-urinary organs, including the seminal vesicles, the gallbladder and the stomach and duodenum.

1. Adami: Colorado Medicine, February, 1914, p. 47.

E. C. Rosenow has experimentally produced ulcers of the stomach in rabbits and in dogs by the intravenous injection of certain strains of streptococci. He has made cultures from gastric ulcers in man, and in two of these ulcers he has found streptococci, taking them from the depths of the ulcer, which leads him to believe in the possibility of such ulcers being infectious in origin. In the animals in which these organisms produced ulceration of the stomach the most common associated lesion was a cholecystitis and beginning gallstone formation.

As gynecologic and abdominal surgeons we must be interested in this pathologic problem in all of its aspects for it is now quite certain that infections may be carried by the blood to the pelvic and abdominal viscera from focal infections in remote parts of the body, as the mouth and tonsils, and, on the other hand, it is equally certain that general systemic infections with embolic lesions all over the body may originate from local foci, more or less chronic or latent in character, in the abdomen.

Rosenow has recently conducted a series of experiments which appear to prove that appendicitis is very often the result of a secondary hematogenous infection from a distant focus like the tonsil.

This conclusion would seemingly be confirmed by the almost epidemic character of acute appendicitis during periods of prevalence of influenza, tonsillitis and grip, so that clinical confirmation of his theory of the etiology of the disease may perhaps be conceded.

The acceptance of this theory of the origin and mode of transmission of infecting organisms from the throat to the appendix by an embolic process and their lodgment and multiplication in the lymphoid tissue of the appendix, for which they may possess a sort of elective affinity, is not in the least incompatible with the contention of this paper, that is, that such a new secondary focus, once established in or about the appendix, may, if not dealt with surgically, be a source of serious and widespread systemic infection; as apparently happened in the instance quoted in this paper.

Lubarsch's most recent studies show that micro-organisms may lead a latent life for a long time until trauma or inflammatory hyperemia makes it possible for them to produce a typical disease. A great number of infectious diseases are of endogenous origin, that is, the micro-organisms were present in the body for a long time before the outbreak of the disease.

Latent, encysted and encapsulated focal infections such as are commonly found about the appendix and fallopian tubes are not to be regarded as free from danger even if no new activity occurs about the seat of the infection.

The clinical histories of such cases are rich with evidence that points to definite damage to remote organs, and to symptoms associated with the circulatory, renal, muscular, nervous and digestive systems which may be attributed to minute though constant hematogenous infections and intoxications from such foci, and which are cured by the removal of the supposedly latent or encysted and partially quarantined focus. One need only suggest to this section a review of our rich experience with the innumerable ills of those women on whom we have operated for old pelvic mixed infections, which were primarily due to the invasion of the oviducts by the gonococcus or streptococcus, followed by colon bacilli and other groups of organisms which have availed themselves of the damaged tissues to gain a foothold. Such patients may not be cured of old organic lesions, of arthritic changes, of established nephritis, etc., but the constant and persistent subinfection may be arrested and further organic changes may be prevented. You have seen many such patients gain weight, lose their pasty complexions and grow rosy and improve in general nutrition and good health after operation. The same improvement may be seen following the removal of an old infected appendix or gallbladder, even though the disease in those organs be secondary to a primary focus in the tonsils or elsewhere.

An acceptance of Rosenow's conclusions as to the hematogenous origin of many if not most of the infections of the appendix leads to the query whether any of the abdominal and pelvic foci from which systemic infections may arise are primary portals of entry, excepting, of course, those of the genital tract.

With hematogenous infections of the kidneys we have long been familiar and we are quite prepared to accept the theory of hematogenous origin for infections of the gallbladder, stomach and duodenum. Foreign bodies in the appendix, though rarely present, may make it vulnerable to the colon bacillus and other intestinal organisms, but its lymphoid elements certainly predispose it to selection when the blood is carrying to it and through it pathogenic organisms from another source.

If then, with the exception of the genital tract, we concede that infecting foci within the abdomen may in many if not in most instances be secondary to some other (primary) focus, a broader and more comprehensive study of such cases is imposed on us.

More thorough and more complete physical examinations must be made to exclude all other possible sources of disease, careful blood studies and cultures are required and the cooperation of other clinicians and of laboratory experts is necessary, for while the elimination of a secondary abdominal or pelvic focus may be accomplished by operation, the primary portal of entry, if one still exists, must be found and eliminated also.

Taking Billings' enumeration of the common systemic results of focal infections of mouth and tonsil origin, and comparing them with such systemic symptoms as may be clinically attributed to foci in the pelvis and abdomen, we find all of them to be common sequelae of such abdominal and pelvic foci. The sub-acute and chronic arthritis of gonorrheal and strepto-coccic origin is common, nephritis and cardiovascular degenerations are frequent and chronic neuritis and myalgias are the habitual and stereotyped complaints of those patients, especially women, who come seeking relief from old pelvic and abdominal infections.

That we as clinicians and as abdominal surgeons must accept the analogy and give greater attention to this phase of the work in our chosen field, that we must acquire a new pathologic conception of the origin and distribution of many such infections, and that we must work in closer cooperation with the bacteriolo-gists and internists will now be quite clear to us all.

More frequent and more exact cultures from foci of infection found in the pelvis and abdomen and more frequent and more exact blood cultures must be made.

Acting on the suggestion of Rosenow we must coop-erate with the bacteriologists in an effort to confirm our clinical convictions. The days of surgical empi-ricism and speculation have passed. Every pathologic theory and belief must be submitted to the acid test of proof.

310 Metropolitan Building.

BIBLIOGRAPHY

Adami, J. G.: Chronic Intestinal Stasis: Autointoxication and Sub-infection, Brit. Med. Jour., 1914, i, 177.

Adami, J. G.: On Latent and Recurrent Infection and on Sub-infection, Jour. Iowa State Med. Soc., 1912, ii, 375-387.

Adami, J. G.: Latent Infection and Sub-infection, THE JOURNAL A. M. A., Dec. 16, 1899, p. 1509, ibid., Dec., 23, 1899, p. 1572.

Adami, J. G., and Nicholls, A. G.: Principles of Pathology, Phila-delphia, Lea and Febiger, 1911, ii, 385.

Auten, F. E.: The Lymphoid Masses; the Part They Play in Infections Gaining Entrance into the Body, Internat. Jour. Surg., 1910, xxiii, 75.

Billings, F.: Chronic Focal Infections and Their Relation to Arthritis and Nephritis, Illinois Med. Jour., 1912, xxi, 261, 274.

Bonney, S. G.: Pulmonary Tuberculosis and Its Complications, Phila-delphia, W. B. Saunders Company, p. 499-501.

Bond, C. J.: A Lecture on the Mucous Channels and the Blood Stream as Alternative Routes of Infection, Brit. Med. Jour., 1913, i, 645.

Casey, J.: Neglected Sources of Infection, Illinois Med. Jour., 1910, xvii, 621.

Canon: Bacteriology of the Blood in Infectious Diseases, Jena, 1905.

Delafield, F., and Prudden, T. M.: Text-Book of Pathology, New York, William Wood & Co., 1914, p. 151.

Digby, K. H.: The Functions of Tonsils and Appendix, Lancet, London, 1912, i, 150.

Davis, David J.: Bacteriological and Experimental Observations on Focal Infection, Arch. Int. Med., April, 1912, p. 505.

Ford: On the Bacteriology of Normal Organs, Jour. Hyg., 1901, v, 1.

Gibbes, H.: Chronic Infections and Their Relations to Internal Disorders, South Carolina Med. Assn. Jour., 1914, x, No. 8.

Jacob, L.: Ueber allgemein Infektion durch Bacterium coli commune, Deutsch. Arch. f. klin. Med., 1909, xcvii, 303-347.

Kocher, Th., and Tavel, E.: Vorlesungen über chirurgische Infektions krankheiten, Jena., 1909, pp. 181-189.

Lane, Sir Arbuthnot: Brit. Med. Jour., 1913, ii, 1125.

Lemaire, Albert: Protective Action of the Liver in Preventing Generalized Colon Bacillus Infection, Arch. de méd. exper. et d'anat. path., 1899, xi, 556.

Lenhartz, Hermann: Die septischen Erkrankungen, In Nothnagel's Spezielle Path. u. Therap., 1903, iii-ii, p. 118.

Manfredi, Luigi: Ueber die Bedeutung des Lymphganglien-systems für die modern Lehre von der Infektion und der Immunität, Virchow's Arch., f. Path. Anat., 1899, clv, 335.

Mayo, C. H.: Local Foci of Infection Causing General Systemic Disturbance, Med. Herald, 1913, xxxii, 370-373.

Neisser, Max: Do Bacteria Penetrate the Intestinal Wall? Ztschr. f. Hyg., 1896, xxii, 12.

Nocard: Influence des repas sur la penetration des mikrobes dans le sang, Semaine Med., 1895, xv, 63.

Rosenow, E. C.: The Relations of Lesions Produced by Various Forms of Streptococcus, Soc. Proc., THE JOURNAL A. M. A., Nov. 29, 1913, p. 2008.

Rosenow, E. C.: Jour. Infect. Dis., 1915, xvi, p. 240.

Southard, E. E., and Canavan, M. M.: Bacterial Invasion of Blood and Cerebrospinal Fluid by Way of Lymph Nodes; Findings in Lymph Nodes Draining the Pelvis, THE JOURNAL A. M. A., Oct. 25, 1913, p. 1526.

Severin, J.: Mitt. a. d. Grenzgeb. d. Med. u. Chir., 1912-1913, xxv, 798-807.

Schnitzler, Julius: Latent Microorganisms, Arch. f. klin. Chir., 1899, lix, 866.

Twort, C. C.: Lancet, London, 1913, ii, 216-218.

Wilson, G.: The Treatment of the Portal of Entry of Systemic Diseases, Tr. Am. Climat. Assn., 1911, xxvii, 257-275.

Wilson, J. C.: Infectious Diseases, Tr. Die Deutsche Klinik, New York, 1905.

Wrzosek, Adam: Latent Infection, Arch. f. path. Anat. u. Physiol., 1904, clxxviii, 82.

ABSTRACT OF DISCUSSION

DR. CARL H. DAVIS, Chicago: During the past two years Dr. Rosenow and I have been working on ovaries in connection with the work which he had done before in the other lines of focal infection. Our results at present are not correlated for publication, but will be published some time this summer. Some of the cases have been extremely interesting.

One patient, an unmarried woman of about 35, had been operated on some five years previously by Dr. Webster.

One ovary was removed and the other ovary resected. A short time after the operation she began to have symptoms even more severe than before the operation. Last year she came back for a second operation and the remaining ovary was removed. Cultures from this ovary gave a pure culture of streptococci in large numbers, and following the operation she had complete relief from the symptoms. Another case shows the probability of a hematogenous infection. It was that of an 18-year-old girl who had marked pelvic pains with a congenital malformation. The cervix was not connected with the vagina and was only connected with the body of the uterus by a fibrous band; yet she had a pure culture of streptococci. Another case worked out more recently, and one in which we will be unable to judge of the results at the present time, was a patient of Dr. Billings. This patient has arthritis, and the teeth and the tonsils and all the other sources had been carefully studied and eliminated. She was operated on by Dr. Webster because of some pelvic condition and an ovary removed. This ovary was studied and a pure culture of streptococci obtained in large numbers. Experimentally Dr. Rosenow was able to pass it through the blood of an animal and produce results in the ovaries of the animal tested.

DR. ALFRED B. SPALDING, San Francisco: Dr. Wetherill suggests to the abdominal surgeon a subject well worthy of consideration. Focal infections, however, work both ways. An infection of a tonsil or the teeth will at times complicate an abdominal infection. A particularly bad streptococcus infection of the tonsil brought this subject very forcibly to my attention some months ago by losing a patient from an acute streptococcus infection of the abdomen following an operation for prolapse of the uterus. The patient was operated on the day after coming to the hospital.

At necropsy there was found a pure streptococcus infection of the bladder, which caused the death of the patient. In reviewing the history it was found that this patient suffered from an attack of tonsillitis some weeks before. She had following this a slight attack of cystitis, which was treated by her physician, and apparently cured. She then came to San Francisco on account of her prolapsed condition. Unfortunately, her history of recent tonsil infection was overlooked.

THE PYLORUS
OBSERVATIONS ON ITS MUSCULATURE

P. E. TRUESDALE, M.D.
FALL RIVER, MASS.

Pyloric insufficiency is a well-recognized barrier to the normal motor function of the stomach. Its causes have hitherto been ascribed essentially to ulcer or cancer. Hypertrophy and atrophy of the musculature of this region as accessory causes have not been recorded, nor have the influences of such changes been considered in the application of surgical principles to the treatment of lesions of the stomach.

Examinations of our resected pyloric specimens for ulcer, fifteen in number, have revealed the interesting fact that such changes do occur and often to a notable degree. The muscular coats of the pyloric end of the stomach and the pyloric sphincter muscle exhibit a distinct overgrowth in the presence of ulcer of the stomach or duodenum. The degree of hypertrophy appears to vary considerably and is presumably governed by the measure of activity on the part of this region of the stomach. Whereas, after gastro-enterostomy, with the stoma functionating well, the musculature of the pyloric end of the stomach, especially the pyloric sphincter, becomes atrophied and atonic. These variations in the musculature of this region are what one would expect to occur in muscle tissue in other parts of the body during continued periods of excessive function and of extended rest. It remains for us to interpret the significance of these transitions. Obviously, they possess a physiologic bearing of considerable meaning, but it is my purpose to deal with their relation to the more common surgical procedures of the stomach.

The failures of gastro-enterostomy have been measurably surmounted by an improved technic and a more judicious selection of cases. Nevertheless, when employed as a single procedure, its career is even now admittedly uncertain, and a study of its disturbing sequences may prove valuable in solving some of the difficulties.

After excision or infolding of the ulcer, our attention has been for the most part centered around the anastomotic opening. Its position in the stomach and jejunum, its dimensions, its angle, its suture line, etc., have exacted the most diligent research. A recent and distinct advance consists in a better choice of suture material as advocated by the Mayos.[1] But this more or less continued variation in the technic of gastro-enterostomy would appear to indicate no small measure of dissatisfaction with its results.

The normal pylorus scarcely admits the tip of one's little finger. The diameter of its sphincter muscle when hardened measures approximately 0.5 cm. It is plastic but rarely does it yield to the dimensions of the average gastro-enterostomy opening. Artificial openings are made large because the small stoma appears to have been ineffectual. A stoma of moderate size would probably be adequate providing its efficiency were not embarrassed by a transition at the pylorus. The structure of interest here is the muscle bundle which embodies the pyloric sphincter. Like the muscular coats of the entire pyloric antrum, it is subject to the variations described above. Whenever the symptoms of pyloric obstruction dominated the clincial picture and the lesion was ulcer, either of the stomach or duodenum, we have observed an overgrowth of the muscle in some cases, reaching 1 cm. and over in diameter. The same specimens showed that the cicatrix of the ulcer played a relatively minor part in the process of occlusion. If these observations

---

1. Mayo, Charles H.: St. Paul Med. Jour., February, 1915.

are confirmed by further study and by other investigators, an additional factor is produced in clearing up the cause of benign obstruction at the pylorus. At the same time we may possess a partial explanation at least of the immediate success of gastrojejunostomy and the gastric disturbances which sometimes recur months or years after operation. This fact in itself, that symptoms often return from six months to two years after gastrojejunostomy, lends weight to the theory of a gradual loss of muscular control at the pylorus following this operation. This deficiency results in a return flow of the contents of the duodenum into the stomach. Findings at secondary operations have confirmed this view. Furthermore, one is inclined to assume that patients who have acquired the greatest degree of muscle hypertrophy at the pylorus, as a class, obtain the most lasting benefit from gastrojejunostomy. The reverse, however, is not necessarily true since it is generally known that the artificial opening and the pylorus may be functionating together, or the pylorus alone in the presence of a stoma, and the patient continues to remain well. However, there is always an unfailing hope on the part of the surgeon who does gastrojejunostomy for ulcer, that in some way the pylorus will close and remain so, for the permanently good results following this blockade are universally recognized.

The cicatrix of an ulcer, especially in the duodenum, must rarely occlude the pylorus. Obstruction elsewhere in the intestinal tract, as from the ulcers of typhoid fever, for example, would be considered very unusual. It is obvious, however, that the edema and engorgement surrounding the ulcer must share to some extent in the occlusion, but this process is transitory and is subject to prompt relief after gastroenterostomy. One of our pylorectomies was done eleven days after gastro-enterostomy for an ulcer mass which, on inspection, I believed to be carcinoma. The second operation revealed a marked improvement in the size and appearance of the tumor due to an amelioration of the inflammatory zone. This is an observation commonly made by other surgeons. Except in the presence of a neoplasm then, permanent obstruction of the pylorus cannot be assured except by division or excision, and to assure the ultimate success of gastro-enterostomy one of these measures would seem to be desirable. Here it may be observed that the success of the Finney operation of pyloroplasty, when practicable, is generally conceded; and that Finney[2] in his operation divides the hypertrophied sphincter muscle completely and permanently. No doubt the logic of this procedure is thus explained.

Whenever the pyloric sphincter is hypertrophied and no lesion can be discovered in the stomach or duodenum, the region of the gallbladder and the appendix should be carefully investigated, for somewhere in the intestinal tract there probably exists a lesion to account for this secondary change which may be due to spasm of reflex origin unless the hypertrophy is congenital, an anomaly which must be rare though not inconceivable. May not the congenital pyloric stenosis now so frequently observed in infants be a partial stenosis and yet a permanent one? Into this class might reasonably be placed an occasional case of "spasm" of the pylorus, considered in infants to be due to improper feeding and not demanding surgical treatment. Most of these patients get well on appropriate food. Is their recovery always permanent? Scudder[3] has shown that the pyloric tumor in infants does not disappear after gastro-enterostomy. The overgrowth of muscle results in permanent closure of the pylorus. If this congenital deformity is one of degree, there follows the natural assumption that an individual who has had gastric discomforts as

2. Finney: Bull. Johns Hopkins Hosp., July, 1902.
3. Scudder: Surg., Gynec. and Obst., September, 1910.

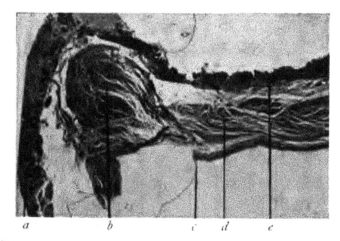

Fig. 1.—Section through normal pylorus of a man, aged 46, who died of a cerebral tumor. From photomicrograph. No lesion was found in the gastro-intestinal tract. *A*, duodenal mucosa; *B*, pyloric sphincter muscle; *C*, peritoneum; *D*, musculature of the pyloric end of the stomach; *E*, gastric mucosa.

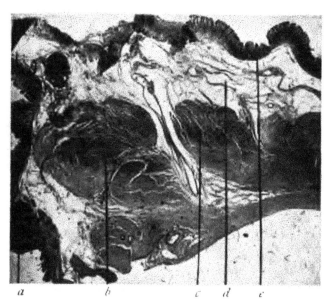

Fig. 2.—Section through the pylorus in the presence of ulcer on the lesser curvature of the stomach 4 cm. from the pylorus. From photomicrograph. Note overgrowth of muscle; *a*, pyloric sphincter muscle; *b*, musculature of the pyloric end of the stomach; *c*, edema of the submucosa; *d*, gastric mucosa; *e*, duodenal mucosa.

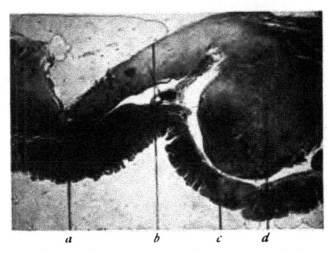

Fig. 3.—Section through pylorus and first portion of duodenum.
From photomicrograph. Ulcer of duodenum; *a*, contraction of peritoneal layer of healed duodenal ulcer; *b*, peritoneum; *c*, gastric mucosa;
d, pyloric sphincter muscle showing marked hypertrophy.

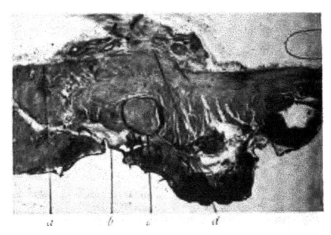

Fig. 4.—Section through the pylorus six years after gastro-enterostomy; *a*, peritoneal layer; *b*, base of ulcer; *c*, atrophied pyloric
sphincter muscle; *d*, omentum and infiltration over site of perforation
seven years ago.

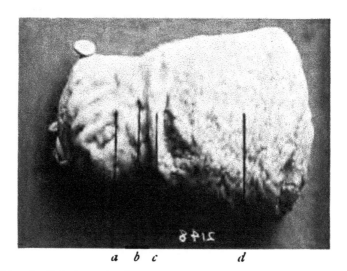

Fig. 5.—Pyloric end of stomach and about 2 cm. of duodenum, removed six years after gastro-enterostomy. Specimen inverted; a, duodenal mucosa; b, small crater of ulcer; c, pylorus—atrophied and widely dilated muscle; d, mucosa of pyloric end of stomach.

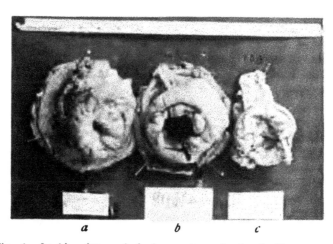

Fig. 6.—Looking into pyloric lumen from duodenal side; a, normal pylorus; b, atrophied, atonic pylorus two years after gastro-enterostomy; c, stenosed pylorus from ulcer.

long as he can remember may have a partial stenosis
that is congenital. The correlation of this lesion in
the adult and the infant was originally based on the
pathologic studies of Maier.[4] Two of our adult
specimens showed a fusiform overgrowth of the
pyloric muscle corresponding to the arrangement of
muscle fibers in the congenitally hypertrophied pyloric
muscle. In one of these cases the history of gastric
disturbance dated to a period as remote as the patient
could remember. "A history of indigestion since the
patient was 2 years of age" was an impressive sentence in the history of a male adult recited in a large
clinic recently where complete records are a feature.
A possible appendix and a thickened pylorus were
the sole evidence that could in any way explain the
history. This is not an uncommon picture, and it is
a disquieting admission that appendicectomy does not
always achieve success.

Hypertrophy of the pyloric sphincter muscle may
have a further significance. McCarthy,[5] in an article
on the "Pathology and Clinical Significance of Stomach Ulcer," writes as follows:

A few cases give previous histories which appear to be
appendicitis. This coincident, if it be a coincident, is well
worth considering, however, as a possible etiological factor. . . . Litthauer has produced ulcers which do not heal
by the production of localized anemia and destruction of
the mucosa. . . . These clinical and laboratory experiences are sufficiently striking to warrant further study and
experimentation in regard to the possible production of
pylorospasm, gastric anemia, hyperacidity and necrosis, or
ulceration of the mucosa.

The hypertrophied pyloric sphincter muscle would
at least appear to be a link in this chain of thought.

Inhibition of the function of the pylorus results in
atrophy of its muscular coats and of the pyloric
sphincter. Whether this interference is due to adhesions of the pyloric end of the stomach to the parietal

4. Maier: Centralbl. f. Physiol., 1887, i, 220.
5. McCarthy: Surg., Gynec. and Obst., May, 1910.

peritoneum and adjacent viscera or to a perfectly functionating stoma, or both, the ultimate change in the musculature will probably be the same. The importance of this alteration is apparent when, in a given case, the degree of muscular atrophy is so marked that the pyloric sphincter entirely loses its function of control. This is illustrated by the findings in one of my cases, a pylorectomy six years after gastro-enterostomy. The anastomotic operation had been done by a master surgeon. When I opened the abdomen, examination revealed the pyloric end of the stomach and first portion of the duodenum extensively involved in adhesion. The first portion of the duodenum could readily be invaginated into the pyloric end of the stomach with the thumb, so atrophied and so atonic was the pyloric sphincter. An examination of the stoma showed some induration and redness around the suture line. Suspecting an ulcer here, I opened the stomach transversely at the antrum. The stoma admitted two fingers readily and the mucous membrane was everywhere normal. The contents of the duodenum poured into the stomach through the dilated pylorus. The stomach was wiped out, the pyloric opening packed with a sponge and the stoma observed. Nothing entered the stomach through this artificial opening. This operation explained the presence of bile in the test meal and an excess of 40 c.c. removed one hour after ingestion. Therefore relaxation of the pyloric sphincter is accompanied by a reversed flow in the duodenum and the duodenal contents enter the stomach through the pylorus as in this case. This phenomenon is in harmony with the laws governing intestinal movements referred to in the researches of Cannon,[6] Starling,[7] and Nothnagle.[8] Cannon reminds us that the presence of acid in the duodenum closes the pyloric sphincter and an increas-

---

6. Cannon: Am. Jour. Physiol., 1901, vi, 251; ibid., 1904, x, 28.
7. Starling: Jour. Physiol., xxiv, 1899.
8. Nothnagle: Beitr. z. Physiol. u. Pathol. d. Darmes., 1884, p. 48.

ing acidity on the side of the stomach causes a relaxation of the orifice. Atrophy and dilatation of the pyloric sphincter, therefore, after gastro-enterostomy is further enhanced by acid in the stomach and an absence of acid in the duodenum. In the presence of this altered chemistry there occurs a progressively increasing muscular relaxation and ultimately an inability on the part of the pylorus to maintain an intermittent closure.

The following cases briefly stated serve to demonstrate the influence of gastrojejunostomy on the pyloric musculature with consequent disturbance of stomach function.

CASE 1.—H. C., an Englishman, aged 46, married, had an unremarkable family and personal history.

Present Illness.—The patient has had stomach symptoms for about twelve years consisting of distress two to three hours after meals and occasional nausea. He rarely vomited. There were no night attacks. Food relief was present. The bowels were constipated. He had decreased 12 pounds in weight. The test meal showed no free hydrochloric acid, yeast cells, but no sarcinae. Large bacilli were noted but no leukocytes or red blood corpuscles.

Operation.—June 27, 1913, a posterior gastro-enterostomy was done for ulcer of the duodenum, also appendectomy. He was symptomatically well for four months, during which time he regained his average weight. Digestive symptoms then began to recur and distress two or three hours after eating. He vomited every morning and has lost 14 pounds in the last six months. Medical treatment gave only temporary relief. Bismuth roentgenoscopy was done by Dr. Dodd of Boston. Writhing of the duodenum was noticed and stasis in the loop.

Second Operation.—April 24, 1914: Adhesions involved the pylorus. The pylorus was patent and atonic. The stoma was adequate and healthy. Von Eiselsberg's operation was done. One year after the second operation this patient is symptomatically well.

CASE 2.—J. M. B., a man, aged 40, married, born in Ohio, had an unremarkable family and personal history.

Present Illness.—In 1907 he was operated on in Columbus for acute perforated ulcer of the duodenum. Eight months later gastro-enterostomy was done. He was well for a year when symptoms, though mild at first, recurred. For the past five years he has had occasional attacks of indigestion lasting from two to three days with distress two to three hours after meals, promptly relieved by soda. He has maintained his average weight. For the past six months he has often been forced to wash out his own stomach, especially at night, because of epigastric distress. There has been no vomitng but occasional nausea. Two weeks before his last operation the stools were noted to be tarry. Long-continued periods of medical treatment only accomplished partial and temporary relief.

A test meal showed excess of 40 c.c. by the tube, free hydrochloric acid, 25; total acidity, 40. Much bile. Bismuth roentgenograms were made by Dr. J. H. Lindsey. The Roentgen-ray diagnosis was of ulcer of duodenum, stasis in the loop, pylorus patent, stoma functioning well.

Operation.—Feb. 20, 1915: Pylorectomy. There were dense adhesions of the pyloric end of the stomach to the parietal peritoneum. The pylorus was dilated and atonic, readily admitting the thumb. The suture line surrounding the stoma was considerably thickened. Suspecting ulcer, I opened the stomach by transverse incision. The stoma admitted two fingers and the mucous membrane was everywhere normal. Bile-colored fluid poured into the stomach through the dilated pylorus while nothing entered the stomach by way of the artificial opening. The pyloric opening was closed by a gauze pack and the stoma then observed. Nothing entered the stomach by this opening. Pylorectomy was done.

Case 3.—H. B., an Englishman, aged 57, married, an upholsterer, had an unremarkable family and personal history.

Present Illness.—Stomach symptoms began about 1907. He was in the Massachusetts General Hospital for observation in 1911. Diagnosis: peptic ulcer. His symptoms consisted of distress two hours after eating, relieved by food or soda. Night attacks were common. Stools tarry. At times constipated.

Operation.—Nov. 13, 1911, a posterior gastro-enterostomy was done for chronic ulcer on the superior surface of the first part of the duodenum; the appendix was also removed. He remained well for two years when the ulcer symptoms began to recur and increased in severity until he was afraid to eat. During this time he had had medical treatment. There has been no nausea or vomiting. His weight has decreased 12 pounds since recurrence of symptoms. A second operation, March 6, 1915, disclosed a dilated atonic pylorus and a healed ulcer. Pylorectomy was done.

In presenting a summary of this paper, I am mindful of the limited number of specimens studied; of the wide variations observed in the degree of overgrowth and atrophy of the pyloric muscle, and of the difficulties of precise interpretation of these phenomena in relation to clinical events. Nevertheless, the evidence thus far obtained demonstrates that:

1. Hypertrophy of the musculature of the pylorus, especially the pyloric sphincter, is found in the presence of gastric and duodenal ulcer.

2. The hypertrophied muscle is a factor in obstructing the pylorus.

3. Atrophy of the musculature of the pylorus is a sequence of gastro-enterostomy.

4. Progressive atrophy of the pyloric muscle often defeats the success of gastro-enterostomy.

5. These changes in the musculature are the result of varying periods of excessive function and of extended rest.

6. Hypertrophy of the pyloric sphincter muscle may be of congenital origin.

1820 Highland Avenue.

For the pathologic specimens and many valuable suggestions in connection with this study, I am indebted to Dr. Annie C. Macrae.

ABSTRACT OF DISCUSSION

DR. FRED T. MURPHY, St. Louis: Dr. Truesdale has centered our attention on the really important section of the stomach, that is, the pylorus. With these microscopic studies of the hypertrophy and atrophy of the muscle layers, I have no observations to present for comparison, but it seems to me to be a very fertile field and we shall certainly try to confirm or disprove these findings. They may offer, I believe, the true explanation for some of the failures which we find in certain postoperative cases, because with the hypertrophy at the time of operation we have obstruction; then, with the final atrophy we have the patent pylorus reestablished and the stomach again empties itself via the pylorus.

One statement of Dr. Truesdale's I greatly appreciated, and that is that the results of gastro-enterostomy without obstruction of the pylorus are at least uncertain. This impressed me as a fair, honest statement of the condition

which the average man finds. It certainly coincides with
what we find at Washington University in St. Louis. In
the cases in which there is frank obstruction at the pylorus,
gastro-enterostomy gives brilliant results, but the idea that
a gastro-enterostomy is a panacea for all lesions of the
stomach seems to me to be absolutely in error, and not in
accordance with the facts which men generally find if they
observe their cases and follow them for sufficient time.

I believe the resection of the ulcer-bearing area is the
logical treatment of these nonobstructing cases. If Dr.
Truesdale had had time I am sure that he would have emphasized the difference between lesions of the stomach and
lesions of the duodenum. It seems to me that today, because
of this failure to differentiate sharply between the lesions
of the stomach and the duodenum, much confusion has arisen.
The lesions of the duodenum either because of the scar contraction or the spasm, tend to obstruct the pyloric outlet,
and therefore gastro-enterostomy gives in every one's hands
relatively good results. In lesions away from the pylorus
and stomach, however, the results are, I believe, as Dr.
Truesdale has stated, at least uncertain.

DR. MAX EINHORN, New York: I saw Dr. Truesdale's
specimens and studied them. He deserves much credit for
doing such important work. From my experience in this
field I think that hypertrophy of the pylorus as a cause of
obstruction is not common. Usually the obstruction is
caused by degenerated tissue, or, in some instances, ulcers
near the pylorus which lead to spasm. In the cases I have
observed there was no hypertrophy yet, but, as the doctor
said, this condition of hypertrophy may develop if there is
a considerable spasm, lasting for a year or longer.

With regard to atrophy, a similar condition may exist too,
as he says; after gastro-enterostomy the pyloric spasm may
disappear, but I have no experience with regard to that.

We meet sometimes with cases in which there are two
things present at the same time—the lack of motility, stag-
nation in the stomach, and patency of the pylorus. The
pylorus can neither close entirely nor can it open well.
This is found not only in malignant disease—although it is
found there most often—but I have found it also in benign
conditions. Thus fibrous tissue interferes with the pylorus
muscle so that it cannot entirely close and cannot entirely
open, and we can make the diagnosis during life. I have
been with patients who had undergone operation and we
found that condition present.

With regard to the function of an organ going on to
definite pathologic changes, I discussed that topic about
eighteen years ago, especially with regard to the circulatory function of the stomach, and I tried to demonstrate
then that a great many pathologic changes are not the cause

of the functional disturbance, but that functional disturbances existing a long time leave the pathologic changes, and that is the same thing that the doctor tries to find now in regard to the musculature of the stomach. This theory was applied years ago with regard to the affection of the spine. At first there is a functional disturbance which leads ultimately to these degenerative changes. I have found similar conditions existing in regard to the circulatory function of the stomach and have tried to demonstrate that in the mucosa of the stomach.

INTESTINAL OBSTRUCTION

ALEXIUS McGLANNAN, M.D.

BALTIMORE

Although aseptic surgery has revolutionized the mortality statistics of acute intra-abdominal diseases in general, the death rate of intestinal obstruction remains almost as high as it was thirty years ago. In the series of 276 cases studied for this report, the mortality was 45.7 per cent. In 161 cases the obstruction occurred in the small intestine, 75 of these patients dying (46.6 per cent.). Seventy-five were cases of large intestine obstructions and have a mortality rate of 44 per cent. In 40 cases the exact position of the obstruction was not given, although it is probable that it was in the small intestine. In the jejunum the obstruction proved fatal in 52 per cent. of the cases.

Much experimental work has been done in the effort to determine the cause of death in intestinal obstruction. This experimental work indicates that the secretion of the duodenal mucous membrane is involved in the production of the essential fatal factor. Hartwell and Hoguet[1] in their experiments show that dehydration is an important element in the fatal outcome of intestinal obstruction, and that in the absence of damage to the mucous membrane of the bowel, this dehydration becomes the most important factor. In pathologic obstruction of the human intestine, met in clinical work, a thoroughly intact mucous membrane is never seen. Early effects of an acute obstruction are manifested in the altered nutrition of the bowel. This is brought about by the interference with the circulation in the wall of the distended coil of intestine proxi-

---

1. Hartwell and Hoguet: Am. Jour. Med. Sc., March, 1912, p. 357.

mal to the point of obstruction. The slow onset of toxemia and its slight degree in a chronic obstruction, may be due to the development of a resistant epithelium with the compensatory hypertrophy occurring in the loop of bowel above the obstruction; or it may be the result of the gradual development of a vicarious function of resistance by another organ.

The original experiments of Draper[2] pointed out in a conclusive manner the existence of a toxic material in the duodenal contents. His later work has confirmed this. Furthermore, the experiments in which obstructed animals were fed minced ileum, indicate the existence of a normal detoxicating function on the part of the epithelium of the lower ileum.

Whipple, Stone and Bernheim[3] have experimented with duodenal obstructions and have proved that if the epithelium be destroyed before the duodenum is obstructed the fatal outcome is avoided.

If the contents of the obstructed duodenum of a susceptible animal be injected into the circulation of an animal of the same species[4] symptoms analogous to those of obstruction occur — vomiting, great prostration with lowered blood pressure, congestion of the kidneys, etc. If the dose of toxin is not overwhelming, the symptoms may be combated by maintaining a supply of fluid by means of hypodermic infusion, and stimulating the failing heart. Epinephrin has been found most valuable for this latter purpose.

The antagonism between epinephrin and the depressing action of the toxin is of interest, because it has been shown that acetylcholin acts as a physiologic antagonist to the suprarenal secretion. Cholin derivatives are prominent in all parts of the body and are easily decomposed, freeing the cholin portion of their molecule. This substance, when hydrolized, yields in

---

2. Draper, J. W.: Experimental Intestinal Obstruction, THE JOURNAL A. M. A., Oct. 21, 1911, p. 1338.

3. Whipple, Stone and Bernheim, Jour. Exper. Med., 1913, xvii, 307.

4. Animals of different species react in divergent ways to the toxin of obstructed intestine. Cats are quite resistant, while dogs, like human beings are extremely susceptible.

turn neurin and muscarin, both depressing poisons, causing vomiting, lowered blood pressure, kidney irritation, etc. Cholin itself belongs to the vagotonic group of drugs, and taken into the body it causes an increased secretion of intestinal juices. One of the striking symptoms of intestinal obstruction is the immense amount of material secreted in the obstructed loops.

All of these facts point to the absorption of a chemical compound of the cholin group of substances, as the underlying essential cause of death in intestinal obstruction.

Toxemia is the real cause of the high mortality of intestinal obstruction as compared with other abdominal diseases. In the present series the causes of death in the fatal cases were the following: toxemia, 75 per cent.; peritonitis, 12 per cent.; postoperative shock, 5 per cent.; miscellaneous, 8 per cent.

Among these 127 cases there were 20 in which the bowel was gangrenous; 14 of these patients died of toxemia, 3 of peritonitis, and 3 others, fifteen, twenty and twenty-six days, respectively, after operation, from pneumonia, tuberculosis and embolism.

The toxemia is combated with great difficulty. Not only are its immediate effects on the heart and vasomotor system dangerous, but secondary effects on the kidneys, liver and other important organs add to the possibilities for disaster. Early recognition and prompt treatment of intestinal obstruction, before the toxemia has developed, offer the only hope we have at present for reducing the high mortality rate. In the present series of cases the average duration of symptoms before operation, in the cured jejunal obstructions, was one and two-thirds days; in the fatal jejunal cases, two and five-sixths days; in the ileum cases the average duration of the cured was three and one-third days, of the fatal, six days. Both sets of cases include some in which the obstruction was probably incomplete. This is especially true of the jejunal series, in one of which death from toxemia occurred although the complete obstruction was relieved in less than four hours after the onset of symptoms, while in another the patient survived, although the operation was performed on the third day. The statistics, however, agree with the acknowledged rule that the higher the obstruction the more rapidly fatal the outcome.

In a previous communication[5] I have discussed the clinical course and symptoms of intestinal obstruction, as occurring in three stages — the stage of onset, of compensation and of toxemia. These stages do not represent any definite period of time, a patient may pass within twenty-four hours through all three and die of toxemia. Gangrene may complicate either the compensatory effort or be present with the toxemia.

In the stage of onset the symptoms are pain, which is usually intermittent and crampy, but may be continuous, nausea and vomiting, with or without constipation or diarrhea. These symptoms come on suddenly and without regard to the ingestion of food. When the bowels move, either spontaneously or as the result of an enema, the pain is not relieved by this action.

Lavage of the stomach may empty that organ of food, gastric secretion or duodenal contents, but without permanently relieving the pain. If, therefore, a patient is suddenly seized with abdominal pain, and an effectual enema combined with gastric lavage does not bring relief from the pain, a diagnosis of acute intestinal obstruction should be made and operation promptly performed.

If there is any hesitation about operating on such slight symptoms, a second lavage should be done after an hour. The presence of duodenal material in the washings at this time, makes the diagnosis certain and operation imperative. In eighteen cases operation was performed during the stage of onset, the diagnosis being made on these symptoms. In every case a mechanical obstruction was found and relieved and all these patients recovered.

In the second stage we have persistent pain, distention, a visible and palpable spastic coil of intestine, visible peristalsis with ladder pattern, local tenderness, etc. In this stage we frequently have gangrene of the bowel and a localized peritonitis at the seat of obstruction. In the third stage the toxemia overshadows the other complications which may be present and becomes the most urgent indication for treatment.

I shall not attempt a discussion of the general pathology and etiology of acute intestinal obstruction as a whole, but shall limit this portion of the paper to a consideration of the postoperative varieties. Of the 276 cases studied, there were 63 in which a previous operation was the etiologic factor. Forty-three patients recovered and 20 died. Of the successful cases 16 followed operation for appendicitis (14 drainage and 2 uncomplicated appendectomies). Twelve were sequelae of various gynecologic operations, and 15 of miscellaneous intra-abdominal operations. Among the fatal cases, there were 9 after appendectomy, all drainage operations, 4 gynecologic and 7 miscellaneous operations. The average duration at the time of operation of the cases resulting in recovery was two and one-eighth days, of the fatal ones, three and one-third days. In sixteen of the fatal cases the patients were operated on in the stage of toxemia.

Nearly 40 per cent. of the postoperative obstructions and 10 per cent. of all cases in this series, follow drainage operations for appendicitis. This is a potent argument in favor of early operation for appendicitis at a time when no drainage is required. Had these patients been operated on thus early, all would have been spared a second operation as a result of which 9 died. About one third of the gynecologic patients had been operated on for inflammatory lesions. In the remaining cases the obstruction was due to involvement of an intestinal coil in the adhesions of some surface left uncovered by peritoneum at the original operation.

Prompt operation in appendicitis and careful covering of surfaces in all abdominal operations, therefore, will afford efficient prophylaxis against postoperative obstruction.

Operative methods will vary with the stage of the disease at which the operation is performed. In the first stage, when there are no complications, the surgeon need only relieve the obstruction. This may be limited to the simple division of the band, or may require a resection and anastomosis for removal of a tumor. Covering in of raw surfaces, or fixation of a particular loop of intestine may become necessary in certain forms of obstruction. In the second stage gangrene of the intestine may complicate the problem. Here the operation performed varies widely with the extent of the gangrene and especially with the general condition of the patient. Practically always these patients are beginning to show signs of toxemia, some have peritonitis, while others have general disease of the vascular system. Almost always they are poor subjects for prolonged operation. Resection and anastomosis is the ideal operation, but often some expedient must be utilized. In the 29 gangrenous cases resection and anastomosis was performed 8 times with 6 recoveries. In 2 of the cases with recovery and one of the fatal cases an enterostomy was made above the anastomosis. Excision of the gangrenous area, leaving the ends of both segments open outside the wound, was done in 12 cases, 10 of which were fatal. A similar procedure with the addition of an anastomosis preliminary to the excision was carried out 4 times, all fatal. The gangrenous loop was extruded in 5 cases. In 4 of these an enterostomy was made above the gangrenous area, one patient recovering.

In the third stage enterostomy may be the only operation that the condition of the patient will justify. At present it appears that enterostomy should be added to any operation done in this stage. Enterostomy either alone or in combination with another operation was performed in 92 cases of this series; 38 of these patients recovered and 54 died. Of the toxic cases without gangrene, enterostomy was done in 77 per cent. of the cases with recovery and in but 41 per cent. of the fatal cases. It is therefore evident that emptying the obstructed loop of bowel has a decided influence on the toxemia, and that enterostomy should be done in all toxic cases, either alone or in combination with other operations, according to the general condition of the patient.

To sum up: The treatment of intestinal obstruction varies with the stage of the disease. Toxemia is the cause of death and is the important factor to be combated in the treatment. In the absence of toxemia the operative procedures are directed toward the removal of the obstructing cause and repair of any damage done the intestinal wall. When toxemia has developed, measures must be devised for combating it, regardless of what may be done in direct attack on the obstruction. These measures are: First, enterostomy for the purpose of relieving the body of material which appears to be the source of the toxemia; second, supplying a large quantity of water, best by hypodermoclysis, in order that dehydration shall not take place, and to stimulate excretion; third, injection of epinephrin intravenously or with the subcutaneous water, to counteract the effect of the toxin on the heart and the blood pressure.[6]

6. The epinephrin solution should be given as follows: After the subcutaneous water is flowing freely, the needle of a hypodermic syringe containing the epinephrin is inserted through the rubber tubing of the transfusion apparatus near the point at which this joins the transfusion needle, and the epinephrin injected into the flowing stream of water. In this way it is carried into the circulation in a fairly concentrated solution without great local reaction.

Toxemia is the constant fatal factor in intestinal obstruction. This explains the slight effect of aseptic surgery on the mortality statistics of the disease. At present we have no certain detoxicating or antitoxic agent, and what slight improvement has been made in the results of treatment must be attributed to earlier intervention. Recognition of the disease in its early stage before the toxemia has developed and prompt operation in this early stage offer the only hope for reducing the high mortality rate of acute intestinal obstruction.

114 West Franklin Street.

ABSTRACT OF DISCUSSION

Dr. John William Draper, New York: We have studied intestinal obstruction from the experimental standpoint for more than ten years and there are certain factors which have come to a focus so definitely as to warrant their presentation clinically. In the first place, I feel that we owe a great deal to Dr. McGlannan's very careful clinical study of this long series of cases. It is the only series in which this has been done, and after all, it is the clinical study combined with the experimental which ultimately will give us the information that we require to save the lives of acutely obstructed patients. First in importance is the aboral portion of the colon. It has a far-reaching bearing on therapeusis. In all of the experimental animals dying from acute intestinal obstruction, the only pathologic lesion demonstrable morphologically was an acute inflammatory condition of the terminal colon. That is almost analogous to the condition seen after the giving of a lethal dose of toxins—for instance, diphtheria—and it suggests very strongly that whatever the toxin may be, the colon plays a very important part in its elimination. This function, however, is restricted to the aboral portion of the colon, if morphologic evidence is to be depended on.

The next point is dehydration, of which the essayist has spoken. Dehydration has been brought to your attention prominently by certain investigators of obstruction who thought that if enough water were introduced into the economy, death would not ensue. There is great variation in individual resistance to toxins, and their dilution by water naturally lengthens life. In the series of experiments we made about two years ago, we showed conclusively by the use of pilocarpin and other drugs that a much greater degree of dehydration might be produced than could be found in animals dying of acute obstructions, yet those animals were perfectly comfortable and showed no clinical signs of sickness whatever. Dehydration is therefore but a small factor in obstructive death. Finally, we have completed another series of experiments, which, while not so conclusive as those previously reported, show amply, in our belief, that the source of the toxin is autogenous rather than bacterial. They coincide peculiarly with the results obtained by feeding kidney tissue after double nephrectomy. The method, briefly, is to feed homologous epithelium of jejunum and ileum to duodenally obstructed animals. While this does not prevent death, it certainly prolongs life. I wish to go on record as believing that these experiments, in conjunction with the studies of Dr. McGlannan, show that the cause of death is not a subinfection of bacterial origin, but rather a true autotoxemia, the unknown poison arising from a perversion in function of the intestinal glands.

Dr. A. McGlannan, Baltimore: In closing I should like to explain my use of the term dehydration in outlining the treatment. I have used it improperly, I see now. I am familiar with the experiments of Dr. Draper, in which the dehydration of animals was produced by salivation, pilocarpin, and so on, and agree with him that the cause of death in obstruction is something much more subtle, and that it is not simple dehydration. I would say, therefore, supply water to dilute toxins. The feeding of the mucous membrane from the bowel below the duodenum is of tremendous interest. My practical experience with it has been none at all. I am hoping to be able to use it in acute intestinal obstruction in the toxic stage, because it may counteract the toxemia, the most important factor to be combated.

THE SIGNIFICANCE OF THE FIXATION OF CERTAIN ABDOMINAL ORGANS IN THE HUMAN BODY

ROBERT C. COFFEY, M.D.

PORTLAND, ORE.

In studying the abdominal cavity from the standpoint of comparative anatomy we find that in man the capsule of the liver has fused with the diaphragm, while in the quadruped the liver is suspended by a mesentery the same as other organs. In man the duodenum is firmly fixed to the right abdominal wall, while in the quadruped it is freely movable. In man the ascending and descending colon and the two flexures are normally fixed to the posterior abdominal wall without the intervention of mesentery, while in quadrupeds the large intestine has a long mesentery and is therefore freely movable. In man the great omentum grows down over the transverse colon and adheres to it. This does not occur in the quadruped. In man the omental bursa is usually obliterated by adhesion of its layers together. Obliteration does not take place in the quadruped. In man the pancreas has been rotated behind the peritoneum and fixed to the abdominal wall. In quadrupeds the pancreas lies between the layers of the mesentery. In the monkey, which is a quadruped with a tendency to stand erect, the pancreas becomes adherent and the duodenum is more firmly fixed than in the original quadruped.

Going more into detail we find that in early fetal life, soon after the beginning of the formation of the alimentary canal, as it elongates, the duodenum, which at first has a mesentery or mesogastrium, turns over to the right carrying, with it the buds of the pancreas.

The duodenum with its mesentery or mesogastrium lies down, so to speak, on the right posterior primitive parietal peritoneum and adheres to it. Thus the duodenum and pancreas become retroperitoneal and fixed. As the colon elongates the cecal end works its way upward and to the right and then down again, locating itself on the posterior and right lateral wall of the abdominal cavity, external to the kidney. The same position is assumed by the descending colon on the left side. At these points the ascending and descending colon and posterior layers of their mesenteries become adherent to the posterior parietal peritoneum, the endothelial surfaces of which become obliterated. Thus the ascending and descending colon not only fix themselves, but put in front of the kidneys the fibrous elements of two extra layers of peritoneum and the vascular and connective tissue structures of the mesenteries of these parts of the colon. The ascending and descending colon and their angles are not only fixed thus by adhesions, but are fixed on a shelf, having an angle of 51 degrees to the perpendicular. This leaves the transverse colon unsupported, except at the flexures and for its own mesentery, until the omentum grows down in front of it and attaches to it. This adds two more layers to its mesentery but does not give it any material support, owing to the fact that primarily the omentum is a sac and the transverse colon is only attached to the posterior layer. Later on, however, often not until nearly adult life, the omental bursa becomes obliterated up to the transverse colon, which gives the colon an extra support from the bottom of the stomach, in the form of a gastrocolic omentum. It is well to bear in mind that the gastrocolic omentum gives no support whatever to the colon until such peritoneal adhesion and consequent obliteration of the omental bursa takes place.

Unfortunately these adhesions do not always take place in man. Very rarely is it true that the duodenum and pancreas fail to adhere to the posterior abdominal wall. Occasionally the omental bursa completely fails to obliterate and permits the center of transverse colon to swing from the flexure without the support of gastrocolic omentum, and occasionally this condition produces serious intestinal stasis. Occasionally the descending colon alone is not fused with the parietal peritoneum and produces, once in a great many cases, a unilateral left floating kidney. The relative infrequency if a left is probably due in a large measure to the costocolic ligament and the gastrosplenic omentum which hold the splenic flexure up much more firmly than the right is held. From 20 to 30 per cent. of human beings have an incomplete fusion of the cecum and ascending colon and its mesentery with the posterior parietal peritoneum. This deficient fusion is of several degrees.

First, the cecum and ascending colon alone may be mobile and very baggy and dilated, swinging from a hepatic flexure which is firmly fixed in its normal position. In a few of this type of cases a false membrane or veil has formed known as Jackson's membrane. This type occurs so frequently and is so slightly mobile that it may be classed as normal.

In the second class of cases the colon has only partially migrated and has attached the hepatic flexure to the front surface of the kidney, leaving the cecum and ascending colon (while the patient is in the erect posture) swinging from the peritoneum on the front surface of the kidney. This peritoneal attachment has been described by Longyear as a distinct anatomic entity under the name of nephrocolic ligament. In some instances the weight of this baggy cecum dropping directly downward pulls the kidney out of position and produces the frequently seen right-side floating kidney. At other times the kidney holds its position, the pendulous colon swings from its attachment as a tube hung over a nail, producing an intermittent obstruction with consequent dilatation of the cecum and ascending colon, resulting in severe intestinal stasis, or the intestine may pull loose, leaving the kidney in its normal position while the hepatic flexure is mobile also. Some of these cases have become partially fixed by a Jackson's membrane.

In the third degree of nonmigration the hepatic flexure attaches to the front surface of the duodenum, when the pendulous baggy cecum with its fluid contents, especially in an individual who has become thin, at times pulls down so strongly on the duodenum as to kink the duodenum at the ligament of Treitz, and also at the junction of the first and second portion of the duodenum. Such a case shows a duodenal stasis with the Roentgen ray, the symptoms of gastric ulcer in the clinical history, and a dilated duodenum at the time of operation. We have seen such patients whose stomach symptoms were entirely relieved as soon as the cecum and ascending colon had been removed. We have seen other cases in which the same relief was obtained by fixation of the ascending colon and the first half of the transverse colon which makes the colectomy unnecessary.

The fourth degree of nonfixation of the ascending colon is seen occasionally and is complete nonfusion in which neither the kidney nor the duodenum have been covered by the mesocolon in which very extreme intestinal stasis existed which was relieved entirely by fixation operation by the method shown in Fig. 1.

In a certain per cent. of human beings there is a nonfixation of both the ascending and descending colon. These are the cases in which the so-called congenital type of enteroptosis occurs, in which both kidneys and all the hollow viscera tend to fall to the bottom of the abdomen, so that when the child reaches maturity the lower abdomen is dilated, the upper abdomen is contracted, the back is straight in an effort of the body to get in under this load and assume the carrying position. We contend that this typical picture of so-called congenital ptosis is due, in nearly all if not in all cases, to a deficient peritoneal fusion, and

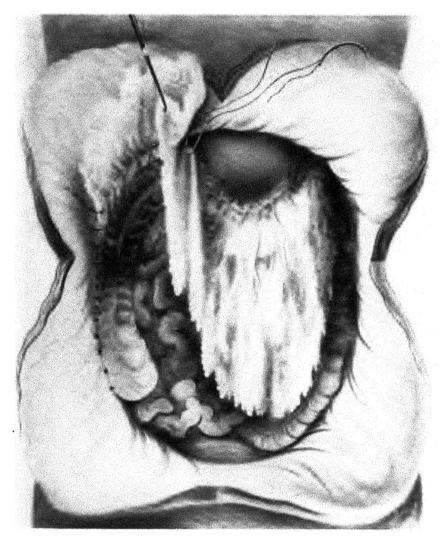

Scheme of operation for anchoring the cecum and ascending colon and suspending the first half of the transverse colon by the great omentum, for a certain form intestinal stasis.

that the peculiar body formation is nature's effort to make the best of a bad job. It is in these cases of nonfusion that all floating kidneys occur. We have been carefully watching for four years and have not found a single case of floating kidney which was not proved on the operating table to accompany a deficient fusion of the ascending or descending colon. In other words, a floating kidney is entirely a secondary condition, which accounts for the fact that the operation for floating kidneys has been considered a failure by most surgeons.

What is the remedy for these defects? In cases of deficient fusion on both the right and left sides, resulting in ptosis with the characteristic body formation, surgery is usually not advised nor indicated. Forced feeding, thereby increasing intra-abdominal pressure, with exercises such as Goldthwaite and also Martin have recommended, will produce the best results. Occasionally the symptoms of a patient suffering from general ptosis are so severe as to require surgical procedure, in which case nothing short of the following operation will do permanent good, namely, the fixation of the ascending and descending colon and the two kidneys, through two separate posterior incisions as described later.

Second, the opening of the abdomen and making a complete partition in the abdominal cavity by stitching the omentum beyond the colon to the parietal peritoneum from one side to the other, thus making a water-tight partition, as we have had opportunity to see at a later operation.

After this operation has been completed the upper abdomen is expanded. Fortunately this very extensive operation is rarely necessary but if any surgery is attempted in the case of general ptosis with the body habitus described by Glenard and Goldthwaite, it is perfectly useless to do less. I have performed this complete operation for general ptosis six times with very satisfactory results, and with much improvement in the patient's health.

A right-side ptosis, however, calls for more frequent surgical interference. A right-side ptosis with a floating kidney accompanied by severe intestinal stasis, pain not relieved by dietary measures, admits of surgical treatment which consists first in making a posterior incision made just as if it were intended to remove the kidney and the first part of the ureter. Before the kidney is disturbed the peritoneum is opened, the appendix removed and the colon sutured to the parietal peritoneum. The peritoneal opening having been closed, the fat capsule of the kidney is opened, a door-flap hinge $1\frac{1}{2}$ inches wide, of fibrous capsule of the kidney is peeled off each side, a piece of the quadratus lumborum muscle as large as the middle finger is split off, two or three quilt chromic catgut sutures are passed through each flap of fibrous capsule, the two from the posterior flap are drawn around back of the separated strip of quadratus lumborum and tied to the corresponding sutures from the anterior, thus using the flaps of kidney capsule like a basket handle around the muscle. The posterior part of the fat capsule is now brought up through the same slit in the muscle and sutured to the front part of the capsule, thus making an additional basket handle of fat capsule.

There are also certain cases of severe intestinal stasis in which the kidney is not movable and in which the hepatic flexure may or may not be movable, giving severe pain in the right side or possibly dragging on the duodenum and producing symptoms of duodenal ulcer, but not relieved by any kind of dietary measures. Such a patient may be entirely relieved by suturing the cecum and ascending and first half of the transverse colon by its omentum to the parietal peritoneum. This, the most frequent operation indicated in the dealing with all defects of peritoneal fusion, is performed as follows: A long right rectus incision is made to expose the entire length of the cecum and ascending colon. If any false bands or membranes have formed they should be cut and a series of purse-string sutures of very fine linen or silk passed but not tied, beginning at the cecum. Each purse-string suture should begin at the true parietal peritoneum to true peritoneum of the colon preferably including a small bight of a longitudinal band. Small bights of the intervening loose tissue should be included. These sutures should be placed every ½ to ¾ inch back toward the normal location of the kidney where the hepatic flexure is fixed. Then the intestine is turned forward and attached by its loose peritoneal connective tissue to the lateral peritoneum to within an inch of the incision and also near to the beginning of the omentum. At this stage of the operation the wall on the median side of the incision is lifted and the omentum sutured to the anterior parietal peritoneum from the median line backwards to meet the other line of sutures (Fig. 1). The omental sutures are of chromic catgut to avoid the danger of extension of a possible infection of the abdominal wound to the line of linen sutures which in two of my early cases kept up a discharging sinus for many months until the linen sutures all came out.

Occasionally a very severe case of constipation is due to the lack of obliteration of omental bursa, and cannot be cured by either dietary or medical means, but is entirely cured after suturing the omentum to the abdominal wall, thereby at once obliterating the omental bursa and holding up the middle of the transverse colon, which prevents the drag of a loaded transverse colon on the flexures.

CONCLUSIONS

1. Prenatal fixation of the pancreas, duodenum, ascending and descending colon and their mesenteries to the parietal peritoneum; of the liver to the diaphragm; of the omentum to the transverse colon; and

the obliteration of the omental bursa, are evolutionary changes which help to fit man for the erect posture are not found in quadrupeds.

2. All cases of floating kidney with general visceroptosis are found in patients whose ascending and descending colon with mesenteries have failed to properly adhere to the parietal peritoneum. Surgical fixation, therefore, of a floating kidney without fixing the colon is not based on sound surgical and anatomical principles, hence the failure of such operations in the past and the necessity for surgical fixation of the colon at the same time.

3. Many cases of intestinal stasis are caused by the disturbed relations of the parts of the intestinal tract resulting from normal fixation of the ascending colon. While most of such cases are relieved by medical means, a few require surgical fixation.

Surgical fixation of the ascending colon should be extended to the suspension of the first portion of the transverse colon by the omentum, for the purpose of preventing harmful angulation at the hepatic flexure. (Fig. 1.)

4. Some cases of persistent stomach trouble are due to the weight of a distended mobile cecum dragging on the third portion of the duodenum, and are relieved by anchoring the ascending colon and suspending the first half of the transverse colon. (Fig. 1.)

789 Glisan Street.

ABSTRACT OF DISCUSSION

DR. MAX EINHORN, New York: I am glad that Dr. Coffey does not commend these operations for enteroptosis. From my experience in enteroptosis, which extends probably over a period of twenty-seven years, I would say that I have not yet seen cases in which an operation was distinctly imperative. Enteroptosis, as such, does not demand surgical intervention. Enteroptosis itself is not of such great consequence nor does it interfere in such degree with the well being of the patients, and we can always do something to relieve them of their symptoms.

It is impossible to fasten each organ in the abdomen. I think we should take it for granted that, having developed from quadrupeds and assumed a standing position, nature probably in the course of the development has already accomplished what we require, and we do not need to worry about it at all or try to imitate those quadrupeds. I do not think they are any better off than we, so that if some organs are not entirely fixed in the abdomen that does not show that they are diseased or that we should change them. A flexible organ can sometimes do its function very well, and if we try to change it we sometimes do harm. That we should bear in mind when we want to interfere.

As to the medical treatment of enteroptosis there are symptoms sometimes requiring correction, and one should try to build up the patient. A great many of these patients with enteroptosis suffer from bad nutrition. They are afraid to eat, and owing to the lack of fat they have those symptoms. If we make them eat and support the abdomen (sometimes such a support is not urgent and they can do without it) we pull the organs up and they improve and we bring about a change in the position of those organs, especially where the enteroptosis has developed after some sickness; the loosening up of the abdominal muscles through this added fat will do wonders. If we build them up, with fat and muscles the organs very often go back of themselves to their natural positions. So in these simple means of nourishing a patient we have our ideal remedy at hand to cure a great many of these patients without surgical intervention.

Dr. ALBERT GOLDSPOHN, Chicago: While the previous speaker was speaking there occurred to me what has frequently been a paradox to me in the feeding question, namely, if these patients do not eat there is something wrong about their gastro-intestinal apparatus causing lack of appetite or fear of the distress which they would afterwards realize. Now, if they are to be permitted to walk about on two feet and not be compelled to go on four, how is the physician to succeed in getting them to eat? And if they are crowded to eat more than they want, is there a proportionate increase in digestion and assimilation following forced feeding?

We all operate for floating kidney rather infrequently. There is probably no operation that I do less frequently than that, and as Dr. Coffey has said, simply fixing the kidney and ignoring the colon, especially when this is done by various uses of the fibrous capsule alone or chiefly, is extremely uncertain in its duration and very unsatisfactory in its results. Dr. Longyear, in suggesting the connection between the kidney and the colon, and speaking of his nephrocolonic ligament, made a step which leads us to think of a possible cause for this dissatisfaction, but I, like many other men, have not been able to trace that ligament. I know, however, that there is a united descent between the kidney and the ascending colon; that the colon is dislocated with the kidney; and I knew that before I had learned of Dr. Coffey's explanation. The technic which I have resorted to, therefore, is chiefly that suggested by Dr. Edward Andrews of Chicago, which consists in making a hammock back of and beneath the kidney out of the fatty capsule and making use of the fibrous capsule only as an adjunct or incidentally. By drawing forward and upward the fatty capsule gathered together on both sides of the kidney, we raise the colon likewise if there is a connection between the two, and by fastening the capsule like the meat in a sandwich, between the muscles in closing the wound by mattress sutures, we can make a fixed and permanent anchorage. This process in the operations that I have performed for floating kidney has been very satisfactory; and I think it coincides with the reasoning and the technic which Dr. Coffey suggests. I think it will be even better to do as he does: enter the abdomen from behind and laterally and anchor the colon and then do this work as he does it on the kidney.

Dr. A. N. Creadick, Portland, Ore.: Dr. Coffey's paper discussed one type of ptosis, namely, congenital, and not the acquired type such as we see in postpuerperal cases, with lost tone of the ventral abdominal wall, a flaccid lower abdomen and the resultant symptoms caused thereby. Let us lay down two or three simple rules for ptosis that will meet with common approval. First, ptosis is established when any supra-umbilical viscus is permanently and wholly below the level of the umbilicus, is then provocative of the usual course of symptoms and requires surgical intervention. No remedy can be applied to this type except the prostrate position or surgical procedure—some such operation as this devised by Dr. Coffey. Second, the "acquired ptosis" patients have some hope in medical treatment of their general asthenic state. The result of such medical treatment is very satisfactory in our hands. A large number of patients are relieved by medical treatment alone. Third. The factors which cause ptosis of the acquired type consist of (a) posture, the loss of the supporting shelf of the spinal column, which Dr. Coffey describes as an angle of 55 degrees from the horizontal; (b) the tone of the musculature of the ventral abdominal -wall and (c) subperitoneal fat. In acquired ptosis the posture can be corrected by gymnastics, which also tone up the abdominal wall as well. (I use the frame devised by Dr. Martin of Chicago, elevating the foot to a window sill, securing an exaggerated Trendelenburg position then requiring the patient to do regular leg exercises.) Hot compresses on the abdomen and forced feeding are useful.

DR. H. O. PANTZER, Indianapolis: I proceed on a theory just the opposite of Dr. Coffey's. Instead of further fixing these organs for cure, I loosen all such angulations, kinks and distortions as interfere with function. In other words, in effect, I choose rather to reestablish the old quadruped condition. I may say that the clinical results are at least equally as satisfactory as those obtained by the fixation methods, which, too, in single cases, are not all we could wish for.

DR. R. C. COFFEY, Portland, Ore.: I never think of operating in these cases until the abdomen is black with blisters which the internist has produced with hot packs during forced-feeding process. The first thing is to have the internist try them out. My colleague Dr. Jones has an institution devoted to the forced feeding treatment. Occasionally there is a case that will not be relieved for mechanical reasons. I know an internist in my city who claims, like Dr. Einhorn, that he can cure them all, but I will say that many of the cases I get come through his hands.

A great many of our best surgeons are inclined to call everything general ptosis. Now Dr. Creadick spoke of acquired ptosis. There is the most definite ptosis seen in the abdomen. The ascending and descending colon have blended in perfectly with the parietal peritoneum and remain in normal position, but the stomach and the middle of the transverse colon have dropped down. This is the most troublesome type of ptosis. It has nothing to do with the subject of my paper and the majority are cured with fattening. Fattening will cure nearly all these cases by increasing the intra-abdominal pressure. The type we are discussing in the paper is an embryologic defect.

CHOLECYSTECTOMY AND CHOLECYSTIC TOXEMIA

W. WAYNE BABCOCK, M.D.
Surgeon to the Samaritan Hospital
PHILADELPHIA

According to the mode of invasion, gallbladder infections may be divided into four types:

1. Portal infection, in which bacteria entering the portal circulation, chiefly from the alimentary tract, escape the bactericidal action of the liver and passing out with the bile, colonize in the gallbladder. This method, described years ago by Adami, has been considered as quite common and is supposed to explain the relationship between appendicitis, intestinal ulceration and other inflammations of the alimentary tract and gallbladder disease.

2. Ascending biliary infection, in which bacteria ascend from the ampulla of Vater through the common and cystic ducts and enter the gallbladder. This process is aided by the reversed mucous currents described by Bond, who showed that carmine particles introduced even as low as the rectum would after a time pass upward against the normal peristaltic current, and be discharged on the surface of the skin through a cholecystostomy opening. Although probably less frequent than other methods, ascending biliary infection occurs in certain inflammations and new growths involving the duodenum.

3. Hematogenous infection, in which bacteria circulating in the general blood stream invade the gallbladder. Rosenow has shown the specific manner in which certain streptococci circulating in the blood,

attack the gallbladder or produce gastric ulcer, and his experiments suggest that many causes of cholecystitis formerly considered of a portal or ascending biliary type are in reality focal hematogenous infections. The well-recognized metapneumonic cholecystitis of young children apparently occurs in this way, as does the infection of the gallbladder in typhoid fever.

4. Contiguity infection, in which the gallbladder is involved by the spread of infection from adjacent organs, as when an adjacent abscess perforates, or malignant or benign ulcer of the stomach or duodenum invades the gallbladder. This is a relatively rare form of cholecystic infection.

Frequence: Infections of the gallbladder are exceedingly common. Next to appendicitis, cholecystitis is the most frequent of all the chronic intra-abdominal infections. In some classes of people, notably obese, middle-aged multiparas, it is more frequent than appendicitis. It is the second great cause of chronic indigestion. Inflammation of the gallbladder often develops during the first and second decades, but as the local symptoms are unobtrusive, the condition usually escapes recognition. After middle age, as the local symptoms become more predominant, the diagnosis of gallbladder disease is made. Thus we have been accustomed to consider it a disease of middle or advanced life.

Persistence: Infections of the gallbladder are exceedingly chronic. It has long been known that typhoid bacilli may continue to multiply for thirty or forty years in the gallbladder. It is now recognized that other bacteria likewise may have persistent growth. The bacteria are found in the center of the gallstone, in the bile, and in the mucosa lining the gallbladder wall. Bacteria found in the center of gallstones and within the depths of the mucosa usually represent more or less remote infections and may be associated with bile that is practically sterile. At present, although most of the patients operated on for gall-bladder disease have reached the fourth or fifth decade of life, a careful study of the history usually indicates that these same patients acquired their infection in the second or third decade. As yet we have not learned to sterilize the chronically infected gall-bladder and the patient once infected may be continuously infected until the gallbladder is removed, or until a violent necrotic form of inflammation destroys the lining of the mucosa and leaves the gallbladder a shrunken, functionless mass of fibro-connective tissue. The temporary relief that follows medical treatment, or a Carlsbad course, prompts the patient and physician to defer operation until advanced pathologic changes have occurred. After a simple drainage operation, the bile clears and the patient is relieved, but the deep infection in the gallbladder wall persists and the symptoms of chronic cholecystitis may later recur. If the symptoms are not of the obstructive type, the patient will usually tolerate them, although not infrequently more radical treatment is demanded.

Symptoms of cholecystitis: Apart from a small area near the neck the gallbladder has no sensory nerves, and distention or inflammation produces no symptoms unless the irritation spreads to adjacent sensitive structures. In operating under local anesthesia, we have repeatedly incised, sutured and crushed the wall of the inflamed gallbladder without pain. Only when traction or pressure affects the ducts, other sensitive organs, or especially the parietal peritoneum, does the patient complain. One should not, therefore, expect local symptoms in inflammations that are limited to the gallbladder proper.

Symptomatically, we would divide chronic chole-cystitis into three stages:

First, a stage marked by more or less remote reflex and toxic symptoms and by the absence of local symptoms. This is the stage of cholecystic indigestion and toxemia and represents a period in which the gallbladder factor is usually unrecognized. It usually continues from fifteen to twenty years before the development of the second stage. In this first stage the mortality under operative treatment should be under 1 per cent.

Second, a stage characterized by the movement of calculi, or by recurrent attacks of acute inflammation. Stones cause paroxysms of pain usually by obstructing the outlet of the gallbladder. The attacks are violent, often follow indiscretions in diet, usually require an opiate, frequently occur at night and last but a few hours. To be differentiated are the acute recurrent attacks of cholecystitis in which no calculi are present. The latter are less violent, usually do not require an opiate, last several days instead of a few hours, and have an onset and termination less abrupt than the colic produced by stone. On exposure, these gallbladders are often considered to be normal, the operator, finding no stones or marked evidences of inflammation, concludes he has made an error in diagnosis. The second stage, or stage of acute biliary paroxysms, is chiefly observed between the ages of 35 and 55 years. The mortality from operative treatment in this stage is from 3 to 5 per cent.

Third, a final stage characterized by acute and dangerous complications, such as empyema, or gangrene of the gallbladder, obstruction of the common bile duct, acute pancreatitis, rupture or perforation of the gallbladder, malignant disease, acute peritonitis, or intestinal obstruction from stone. These complications marking the third stage of cholecystitis are most frequently observed between the ages of 45 and 75. One of our patients was 80 years of age, seven were over 70. Unfortunately, a large proportion of patients reach the third and dangerous stage of cholecystic infection before coming to operation. That one fourth

of all the operated patients of a well-known surgeon
should have had associated disease of the pancreas is
a sad commentary on medical delay. The occurrence
of the third stage of cholecystitis is a reproach to
our medical art, and indicates an average procrastina-
tion in the effective treatment of cholecystitis of about
twenty years. Rather unusually, of course, we meet
with exceptions. Thus during the past year I have
seen one girl of 14 years with over three hundred
gallstones, acute pancreatitis and fat necrosis; and a
boy of 15 years with twenty-eight gallstones, localized
peritonitis and a gangrenous gallbladder 7½ inches
long. The mortality in this stage of cholecystitis probably averages over 20 per cent. The relief from many
reflex and secondary symptoms of early biliary infection, the prophylaxis of gallstones and of the dangerous
complications of cholecystitis lie in the effective treatment of the first stage of cholecystitis, and therefore the recognition of this stage deserves special
consideration.

The evidence of cholecystitis of the first stage is not
found in a physical examination of the upper right
quadrant of the abdomen, but is to be determined by
deductive reasoning. The history of the patient usually
reveals a cause of infection which has a relationship
to the development of certain reflex toxic, or secondary
infectious processes that experience has shown frequently to express cholecystitis. These may be
grouped as follows:

(a) Digestive: Most common are the reflex digestive
symptoms. Fulness and distress after eating, with
sour bitter eructations, belching, and more rarely
vomiting are usual. There may be a constant foul
taste in the mouth, which at once disappears when
the gallbladder is drained or removed. The dyspepsia
is of the "qualitative" type, rather than the "quanti-
tative" dyspepsia of ulcer; that is, attacks of indigestion often follow certain articles of diet, such as

shellfish, cheese, boiled dinners, fried foods, pastries, corn, and the like, and may not be influenced by the amount of food eaten. The patient will often mention an idiosyncrasy toward certain foods. The inability of a patient to handle certain staple articles of diet should suggest biliary disease. It is perhaps the most common condition that causes a patient to report periodically to a physician for relief from attacks of so-called biliousness or indigestion. The attacks are usually relieved temporarily by fasting, dieting, by alkalies, or by a saline or calomel course.

As to the differential diagnosis, transient, often nocturnal, attacks of indigestion in an obese, middle-aged woman precipitated by a dietetic indiscretion and requiring a hypodermic injection for relief, are rarely due to other causes than gallstones. With the history of such preceding attacks, a very violent and persistent attack suggests empyema, or gangrene of the gallbladder; while an attack of superlative severity with shock and epigastric distention and tenderness usually means a pancreatitis. As contrasted with gastric or duodenal ulcer an attack of gallstones lasts a few hours, is most abrupt and severe; an acute cholecystitis a few days and is less severe; while an ulcer attack usually lasts for several weeks and is the least severe. Between the paroxysms from stone or acute cholecystitis, which may be months or weeks apart, the patient usually has a greater degree of dyspepsia than is found between the exacerbations of ulcer. In ulcer, feeding may give temporary relief, "food ease"; while distress accompanies an empty stomach "hunger-pain." In cholecystitis and stone, food exacerbates and vomiting relieves the pain.

(*b*) Intestinal symptoms: The intestinal symptoms of cholecystitis are as yet not fully understood. The continuous discharge of bacteria laden bile into the intestinal tract may give rise to the so-called intestinal indigestion, and in some instances to the symptom of intestinal toxemia, so graphically described by Mr. Lane. It is possible that some of these patients have been given a measure of relief by the removal or elimination of the colon, not because the cause was removed, but because the absorptive surface of the intestine was reduced. There is an association between cholecystitis and appendicitis, the appendix either infecting the portal system and gallbladder, or being coincidentally infected by a common cause. Wohl has reported that in 50 per cent. of our cases in which the removed appendix was also studied, there was evidence of appendicitis.

(c) Peritoneal symptoms: Peritoneal symptoms result from acute inflammation or secondary adhesions. The forms of localized or diffused peritonitis that may result from the later stages of gallbladder infection require little special discussion. Attention should be directed, however, to the frequent error in mistaking cholecystitis for appendicitis. An enlarged inflamed gallbladder, with only a small area of the fundus projecting below a Reidel lobe of the liver, frequently produces recognizable peritoneal inflammation only when the exposed fundus comes in contact with the sensitive parietal peritoneum, and this frequently is directly under McBurney's point. In nearly every such instance which we have seen, the examiner, overlooking the less distinct and less sensitive area of resistance which spreads down from the right costal border, has concluded that acute appendicitis was present.

(d) Arthritic and muscular complications: Subacute or acute metastatic joint infections are frequently observed in chronic cholecystitis. Often these symptoms improve after cholecystectomy. Chronic joint changes of the type of arthritis deformans are also observed. Myalgic pains are exceedingly common.

(e) Cardiovascular symptoms: Few patients pass to the third stage of cholecystitis without some evidence of cardiovascular disease. Endocardial and particularly myocardial changes seriously increase the risk of anesthesia and of operation in long-standing gall-bladder disease. To some degree pathologic changes of the arterial wall also have their origin in cholecystic infections. Cardiovascular symptoms may greatly improve after operations on the gallbladder.

(*f*) Respiratory symptoms: We have been impressed by the surprising relief from paroxysmal cough and asthma that may follow cholecystectomy, or cholecystostomy, and we have operated for these symptoms alone. Two of our patients who had been unable to sleep except in a sitting posture for five and seven years, respectively, found they could recline with comfort after the operation, and the asthma and cough disappeared. After a period of relief for some weeks, however, the symptoms recurred. It would seem that cholecystic toxemia is a factor in some of these cases.

(*g*) Cerebrospinal symptoms: In cephalalgia, neuritis and some of the neuroses relief may be obtained by operating on the gallbladder. In the so-called bilious sick headaches we have observed relief after cholecystectomy, and in one violent case we operated for this symptom alone, with relief. In this case the symptom was a sequence to typhoid fever. In certain of the prematurely worn women of middle age, who constantly complain of indigestion, bloating, constipation and a multitude of aches, pains and surface paresthesias, there has been something of a mental transformation after the removal of a chronically infected gallbladder.

(*h*) Fever: Fever without other symptoms may result from cholecystic infection. The bile may be free from pus, the gallbladder bluish and nearly normal in appearance. The fever disappears with the removal of the gallbladder. One of our patients with no local symptoms had been treated in hospitals for months for an apparently causeless continuous fever, that immediately subsided after the excision of what seemed like a normal gallbladder.

(*i*) Eye symptoms: Eye symptoms are not infrequent with biliary disease. At times we find the oculist promising relief from the digestive symptoms of cholecystitis by the application of glasses, or, again, vainly attempting to control a vacillating series of refractive or muscular abnormalities.

DIAGNOSIS

The diagnosis of cholecystitis after opening the abdomen is not always easy. We depend on one or more of the following abnormal conditions:

1. Alteration in the color, size or consistence of the walls of the gallbladder. A milky or whitish gallbladder is diseased, but many translucent, bluish gallbladders are also diseased.

2. Adhesions or other evidence of pericholecystitis. Often the liver adjacent to the gallbladder shows evidence of chronic perihepatitis by whitish plaques or connective tissue trabeculation.

3. Enlargement of tributary lymph nodes: Attention has been especially directed by W. J. Mayo to the lymph nodes. The palpating finger is introduced into the foramen of Winslow and the nodes near the junction of the cystic and common ducts examined. While such lymph-node enlargements usually indicate cholecystic infection, they may also occur from pancreatic or duodenal disease. Absence of enlargement unfortunately does not negative cholecystitis. At times we have observed the absence of adenopathy in purulent or gangrenous as well as in catarrhal cholecystitis.

4. Alterations in the bile contained within the gallbladder: Normal bile is of a clear golden yellow color; turbid, purulent, dark green, tarry bile, or bile containing crystals, sand or calculi, indicate cholecystitis. Colorless mucus indicates cystic-duct obstruction and a mucocele. For diagnostic aspiration, to avoid leakage, should the gallbladder not be removed, a fine needle should be introduced into the gallbladder through a thin layer of overlying liver substance.

5. Alterations in the mucosa: Papillary denudations producing the finely speckled or strawberry gallbladder, papillary outgrowths, infiltrations of the mucosa as well as the grayish, greenish or blackish wall, or sloughs seen in empyema or gangrene, indicate varying grades of gallbladder disease.

PROGNOSIS

Cholecystitis may be alleviated by dieting, alkalies, salicylates, vaccines or a saline or Carlsbad course. It is more surely curable by the operative removal or obliteration of the mucous lining of the gallbladder. Most patients who finally come to operation have had some degree of relief from dieting, or various medical measures. In a woman who, for six years, following typhoid fever, had suffered from indigestion, headaches, myalgia, bromidrosis and foul taste, the symptoms almost completely disappeared after a course of typhoid vaccines. Except in the third stage of cholecystitis which brings an immediate danger to life, operation is usually delayed or considered unnecessary. At present, surgery, which is about the only permanently effective therapeutic measure against cholecystitis, is about twenty or thirty years behind the pathology of the disease, usually ignoring the early stages of inflammation and cholecystic toxemia, permitting years of morbidity and crippling tissue changes to supervene, and only intervening when a violent local reaction drives the patient to the surgeon.

OPERATIVE TREATMENT

Anesthesia: An anesthetic may increase the danger of operation on the biliary tract by depressing the cardiac and respiratory systems, adding to the preexistent toxemia, inhibiting elimination, and by producing straining movement, violent respiratory action and rigidity of abdominal muscles, that so embarrass the surgeon as to invite dangerous technical errors. At the Samaritan Hospital during the past three years, one patient with a perforated gallbladder and an upper abdominal peritonitis, was asphyxiated by profuse, regurgitant vomiting, while under spinal and narcotic anesthesia. In a second patient with myocarditis, cholecystitis and acute peritonitis there was a fatal respiratory cardiac failure. A third similar fatality occurred under the administration of ether. We have been able to reduce the mortality by substituting local anesthesia for patients who are bad risks. The local anesthetic solution is used very freely, 1 per cent. of novocain being employed for the skin and subcutaneous tissues, and a 0.25 or 0.5 per cent. solution being employed for the muscular, fascial and peritoneal layers. A free injection of such weak anesthetic solutions seems not only harmless but often beneficial, acting like a hypodermoclysis in assisting elimination. If the patient's general condition permits, a moderate supplemental narcosis produced by morphin-scopolamin is used. Especially in the very old, the very toxic or asthenic with empyema or gangrene of the gallbladder, or perforation and peritonitis, do we prefer local anesthesia. For patients in better physical condition, we prefer spinal anesthesia because it does not interfere with elimination or increase preexisting toxemia, and at the same time gives far better relaxation than ether does. It is dangerous for operations on the gallbladder in obese elderly patients who are toxic and have serious myocardial change. Rectal anesthesia, from its especially intense action on the liver, should be avoided.

Incision: A simple transverse incision made along a line slightly below the level of the ninth rib is valuable when operating under local anesthesia, especially if the gallbladder is large and there is marked muscular rigidity. In such a case the gallbladder and liver margin may be made to protrude from the opening and retraction and the introduction of pads within the abdomen are unnecessary. It is especially adapted for cholecystostomy, although occasionally a chole-cystectomy may very conveniently be done. For the former operation a shorter incision may be employed, the different layers being divided along the same line. To give a better exposure of the ducts, a triangular flap incision, as suggested by Perthes, may be used. A right transrectus incision is made from the ensi-form directly downward for 3 or 4 inches, from the lower end of this vertical incision a transverse inci-sion is made to the right to a point just below the right costal margin. The vertical part of the incision is carried through the rectus to the posterior sheath and guided by the finger introduced behind the rectus fibers; two or three sutures of catgut are placed above and below the line of the transverse incision in such a manner as to fix the rectus muscle to the overlying aponeurosis, so that the divided muscle will not retract. The muscular and aponeurotic layers are now divided along the line of the transverse incision and the trian-gular flap thus formed turned upward and outward over the chest wall. The peritoneum and preperito-neal fascia are now divided along a line parallel with the costal border and about one-half inch distant from it. To avoid the objectionable right-angle incision of the skin, I have modified Perthes operation by substi-tuting a simple oblique skin incision which is made parallel with the costal border after the plan of Kocher.

Alexander Don, to obtain a greater exposure and to avoid injury to the intercostal nerves, extends the vertical portion of the incision down to the level of the navel, and curves the transverse portion of the incision upward and outward toward the right axilla. The rectus muscle is completely freed and divided below and the posterior sheath of the rectus and peri-toneum divided along the same lines as is the skin.

In patients with relaxed or thin abdominal walls a simple vertical transrectus incision often serves very well.

Cholecystectomy: In the first stage of cholecystitis, cholecystectomy is the preferred operation. It is the most effective method of treating the protean manifestations of the disease. The patients are usually under middle age, are not very obese and come to the operating table in good physical condition. With a perfect technic the operation in this stage should be a safe and satisfactory one, but unfortunately there are serious technical dangers always present in doing a cholecystectomy; an unfortunate snip of the scissors, a careless needle puncture or an imperfect ligation, is all that is required to place the patient's life in jeopardy, and these accidents have caused many surgeons to resort to ostomy when an ectomy would be the better operation. Even so skilful an operator as Moynihan reports three cases in which an hepatic or common duct was wounded. In my first ectomy, a case in which there were extensive intra-abdominal adhesions, the divided cysticus was imperfectly occluded and a secondary fatal leakage of bile into the peritoneal cavity occurred. In a recent case the gallbladder was distorted and displaced by adhesions, and on closing the peritoneal edges over the gallbladder bed, biliary leakage, evidently from a punctured displaced hepatic duct, occurred. The stitches were removed and drainage was instituted, with recovery. We have had three other cases of accidental duct injury or imperfect ligation of the cystic duct during cholecystectomy. These accidents are less frequent when the operation is performed in the first stage of cholecystitis. Since the first case we have now had 114 ectomies during the first stage of cholecystitis without operative mortality. In this stage the gallbladder is usually best removed from within outward, after the method so well illustrated by the Mayos. The cystic duct should be doubly ligated, mass ligatures should be avoided, as should anything which may serve to distort or obstruct the ducts. The cystic artery should be individually tied.

Wide flaps of peritoneum should be separated from the gallbladder to cover the denuded area left under the liver. If there is any question as to absolute hemostasis or duct occlusion adequate drainage should be employed, so arranged or anchored by fine catgut that it cannot be displaced. In most of our ectomies we have been able to avoid all drainage. In cases of the second or third stage when the gallbladder is distorted or imbedded in adhesions, it may be safer to remove the gallbladder from without inward. In this way, by hugging the gallbladder very closely, there is less danger of damaging the hepatic or common duct. In case the adhesions are very marked, the method of Kehr of first splitting down the interior surface of the gallbladder at least into the cystic duct, is an advantage in determining the relationships of the parts.

Cholecystostomy: External biliary drainage, considered by the late Dr. Maurice Richardson only ten years ago, the one established therapeutic fact in biliary surgery, has a progressively lessening sphere of usefulness. Its use should be largely restricted to the third stage of cholecystitis for cases of empyema, perforation, gangrene, pancreatitis, advanced peritonitis or duct involvement, associated with such grave systemic changes due to age, toxemia or exhaustion, that only the simplest of operative procedures are warranted. It also should be used when technical limitations indicate that an ectomy will be dangerous. Under certain favorable conditions by performing cholecystectomy, we have been able to avoid drainage even in cases of empyema, gangrene of the gallbladder and acute pancreatitis. As a rule, the virulence of the bacteria found in empyema or gangrene against the skin and subcutaneous tissues is less than that of the bacteria found in purulent forms of appendicitis.

As cholecystectomy is the great measure of prophylaxis, it should be performed more frequently and much earlier and should have a progressively lower mortality than cholecystostomy.

If reasonably safe and feasible the appendix should also be removed in operating for cholecystitis. Despite certain results of animal experimentation, clinical evidence indicates that a patient is better off without than with a chronically infected gallbladder.

The mortality of cholecystectomy is due to: 1. Poor judgment in selecting patients with acute febrile and septic conditions, or patients greatly debilitated by age, chronic toxemia or complete and continued external drainage of bile. This latter class who have what we may term "cachexia-choleoprivia" bear operation very badly, readily falling into a condition of fatal shock irrespective of the operation or anesthetic employed. For them a simple Witzel enterostomy should first be done under local anesthesia and the bile shunted from the fistula into the bowel by a small rubber tube. The final operation should be delayed until the cachexia, due to the loss of bile, has been overcome.

2. Technical errors: Leakage of bile into the peritoneal cavity may result from the cystic duct having been imperfectly tied, or the common or hepatic duct torn, incised or punctured. In the case of bile leakage, if the general peritoneal cavity is not sufficiently protected by drainage and tamponade, a dangerous or fatal peritonitis may result. I have been impressed by the danger of (a) doing cholecystectomy in a private house where adequate light and sufficient exposure cannot be obtained; (b) separating the overhanging neck of the gallbladder without observing great care in hugging the gallbladder proper to avoid the adjacent communis; (c) puncturing the hepatic duct. The gallbladder may lie obliquely so that the hepatic duct is in the peritoneal fold to the side of the neck of the gallbladder, where it may be damaged in suturing over the gallbladder bed; (d) relying on insufficient tamponade for drainage in the presence of a biliary

leak. In all cases, as an indicator, we place the end of a gauze sponge against the stump of the cystic duct, which is not removed until the end of the operation. Should this show staining by bile, we immediately reopen and control or isolate the area.

In a personal experience of 270 operations on the gallbladder and ducts, fifty-seven ectomies were done before 1912 with ten deaths, a mortality slightly over 17 per cent. In thirty-eight ostomies before 1912, there were three deaths, a mortality of 7.8 per cent. In 121 ectomies performed since 1912, there were two deaths, a mortality of 1.6 per cent. In forty-two ostomies since 1912 there were four deaths, or about 9 per cent. mortality. Before 1912, gangrenous and suppurating gallbladders were usually removed; now they are usually drained under local anesthesia. As having even a greater influence on the mortality is the stage in which the operation is done. In 114 cases of ectomy in the first stage of cholecystitis, irrespective of date or technic, the mortality was 0.88 per cent. In 101 operations in the second stage, sixty-seven being ostomies, there were four deaths, a mortality of 3.9 per cent.; while after fifty-four operations in the third stage of cholecystitis, there were eighteen deaths in which the operation or biliary condition was a factor, a mortality of about 32 per cent. Thirty of these patients had acute gangrenous or suppurative cholecystitis, seven an acute pancreatitis with fat necrosis. Twelve had primary or secondary operations for duct obstruction, fistula or duct or intestinal anastomosis. In only one patient was carcinoma observed, and this involved the ducts. In two cases, intestinal obstruction from gallstone existed. In another case an intestinal perforation had been produced. One death was from diabetic coma and one from pulmonary embolism. It is evident that the stage of the disease is more important than the type of operation in determining the mortality.

SUMMARY

We consider inflammations of the gallbladder as bacterial infections of childhood or early adult life, as progressing for years, during which time secondary metastatic, toxic or reflex symptoms only are observed; as later having a second stage in which there are attacks of colic due usually to the presence of gallstone; as having usually after twenty or thirty years a third stage of serious complications, such as duct obstruction, pancreatitis, perforation, abscess or gangrene. We consider surgery as working, for the most part, far behind the pathology of the disease, and believe there is wide need for earlier intervention, so that the patient who starts at the age 12 or 15 with cholecystitis and dyspepsia may not at 35 have gallstone colic, and may not at 65 succumb to cholecystic gangrene or pancreatitis. We consider external biliary drainage as a rule undesirable, except in the late or complicated cases, an early cholecystectomy the operation of choice. Unfortunately, technical dangers make uniform success after cholecystectomy uncertain in the hands of the average surgeon. Despite this, the mortality of cholecystectomy in the first stages of cholecystitis is much less than cholecystostomy in the last stages of this disease, so that the results of a surgeon may depend more on *when* he operates than *how* he operates. The morbidity depends on *how* he operates.

2033 Walnut Street.

ABSTRACT OF DISCUSSION

Dr. Robert C. Coffey, Portland, Ore.: In dealing with third stage, acute stage cases, in which there is an infected gallbladder, I wish to emphasize conservatism. It is often the case that these gallbladders may be enucleated by a simple incision of the peritoneum and peeled out practically without bleeding at all. There are some cases, however, in which this is not advisable. I refer to acute and violent septic cases. The point I wish to emphasize particularly is that this area must be quarantined properly. Expose the field thoroughly and place a large pack of gauze wicks laid straight down around the gallbladder, and around these wicks several layers of rubber tissue. Open the gallbladder, sponge out the fluid and insert a piece of gauze into the gallbladder. That is all that is necessary. It will take approximately five minutes. Many are gangrenous without widespread infection and it is quite safe, in these, to enucleate the gallbladder, which I say is easily done without hemorrhage at all. The gauze wicks of the pack are removed after six days and the rubber tissue in two weeks. In some instances it will be necessary to remove the gallbladder at a later operation.

Dr. W. Wayne Babcock, Philadelphia: In the young no drain may be required after ectomy. There is less danger of skin infection from removal of the gangrenous or suppurating gallbladder than from removal of a badly infected appendix, and therefore as far as wound infection goes, less need for wound drainage. When the patient is in good general condition, we may, therefore, in selected cases remove the badly infected gallbladder, close without drainage, obtain primary union, and a remarkably quick recovery. One patient went home a week after the removal of a gangrenous gallbladder. But as a rule, and especially if the patient has reached middle age and the gallbladder is gangrenous, ectomy is dangerous. In these cases we use local anesthesia, make a simple transverse slit, put in a drain, and sometimes even operate without removing the patient from the bed. The sloughs of the gangrenous gallbladder will be expelled with relative safety, while the removal of the gallbladder, by opening many lymph spaces, may be followed by rapid sepsis and overwhelming toxemia.

LIST OF FELLOWS OF THE AMERICAN MEDICAL ASSOCIATION REGISTERING IN THE SECTION ON OBSTETRICS, GYNECOLOGY AND ABDOMINAL SURGERY

The following is a list of Fellows of the American Medical Association who, at one or more of the last five sessions, have registered in the Section on Obstetrics, Gynecology and Abdominal Surgery, together with Fellows who are subscribers to the transactions of the Section for 1915. The figure following the name indicates the year in which the member registered (0 indicating 1910, 1, 1911, etc.). T indicates a subscriber to the transactions. Any errors which may have occurred should be brought to the attention of the secretary of the Section.

Abbott, Chas. N., Chippewa Falls, Wis. 3.

Abbott, Geo. E., 161 N. Los Robles Ave., Pasadena, Calif. 1.

Abrams, Edw. T., Dollar Bay, Mich. 9, 0, 3, 4.

Adair, Fred L., 820 Donladson Bldg., Minneapolis. 3.

Adams, C. T., 5701 Girard Ave., Philadelphia. 9, 2.

Ahrens, A. H., 920 Rice St., St. Paul. 3.

Alderson, J. C., 311 Jefferson St., Wausau, Wis. 3.

Alexander, A. F., 379 Union Ave., Paterson, N. J. 7, 9, 1, 2.

Alexander, Robt. J., Amicable Bldg., Waco, Tex. 4.

Alleben, J. E., 402 Masonic Temple, Rockford, Ill. T.

Allen, Frederick B., 147 N. Main St., North Wales, Pa. 2.

Altman, J. T., cor. Church and Vine Sts., Nashville, Tenn. 4, 5, 6, 0, 2.

Anderson, A. E., Griffith McKenzie Bldg., Fresno, Calif. 5.

Anderson, Winslow, 1065 Sutter St., San Francisco. 0, 1, 5.

Andrews, Leila E., 404 Colcord Bldg., Oklahoma City, Okla. 4.

Anneberg, A. R., Golden West Hotel, Carroll, Iowa. 5.

Anspach, Brooke M., 119 S. 20th St., Philadelphia. 9, 2, 3, 4.

Apjohn, Henri, Box 94, Yuma, Ariz. 1.

Appel, Theo. B., 305 N. Duke St., Lancaster, Pa. 3.

Applegate, J. C., 3540 N. Broad St., Philadelphia. 2, 4.

Arnold, J. O., 2503 N. 18th St., Philadelphia. 7, 9, 2, 4.

Arnett, Jas. H., 2540 N. 11th St., Philadelphia. 4.

Arthur, Mattie L., 407 Paxton Blk., Omaha, Neb. 1.

Ashton, Wm. Easterly, 2011 Walnut St., Philadelphia. 2, 4.

Ashum, David W., Eau Claire, Wis. 3.

Auge, Emily G. Whitten-, 2734 Wharton St., Philadelphia. 4.

Bachmann, Geo. W., 330 Central Park, Rochester, N. Y. 4.

Bacon, Charles E., 730 Kingsley Drive, Los Angeles. 1.

Bacon, Charles S., 2156 Sedgwick St., Chicago. 4, 5, 6, 7, 8, 9, 0, 2, 3, 4.

Bacon, Knox, 1118 Summit Ave., St. Paul. 3.

Baer, Jos. L., 4755 Forrestville Ave., Chicago. 4.

Bailey, Harold C., 269 Lexington Ave., New York City. 2.

Bainbridge, Wm. S., 34 Gramercy Park, New York City. 4.

Baird, Alvin W., Medical Bldg., Portland, Ore. T.

Baldwin, J. F., Grant Hosp., Columbus, Ohio. T.

Baldy, John M., 2219 DeLancy St., Philadelphia. 0, 2, 4.

Ballard, W. R., 205 Ridotto Bldg., Bay City, Mich. T.

Balleray, G. H., 115 Broadway, Paterson, N. J. 5.

Ballin, Max, 367 Woodward Ave., Detroit. T.

Barbat, J. Henry, 275 Post St., San Francisco. T.

Barnard, E. P., 119 S. 19th St., Philadelphia. 4.

Barnes, C. S., 35 S. 19th St., Philadelphia. 9, 2, 4.

Barnes, S. S. P., 311 E. Main St., Massillon, Ohio. 9, 1.

Barney, Delbert, 55 N. Washington St., Wilkes-Barre, Pa. 2.

Barney, N. Eugenia, Sterling, Colo. 1, 5.

Barnhart, Wm., 318 N. Mathews St., Los Angeles. 1.

Barrett, C. W., 561 Stratford Pl., Chicago. 4, 6, 9, 0, 3, 4.
Barrett, Fred'k, Giibert, Minn. 3.
Bartlett, C. W., 70 North St., Bennington, Vt. 4.
Bastian, Jos. W., 915 Washington St., Wilmington, Del. 4.
Battey, H. I., 604 Atlanta Nat. Bk. Bldg., Atlanta, Ga. 3.
Baxter, Stephen H., 2000 Hennepin Ave., Minneapolis. 3.
Beach, Edw. W., 5401 Spruce St., Philadelphia. 4.
Beattie, T. J., 1203 Waldheim Bldg., Kansas City, Mo. T.
Beck, Henry E., 720 16th Ave., Moline, Ill. T.
Bell, J. N., 1149 D. Whitney Bldg., Detroit. 0, 3, 4.
Benjamin, A. E., 2222 Blaisdell Ave., Minneapolis. 6, 9, 0, 1, 2, 3, 5.
Bennet, E. H., Main St., Lubec, Maine. T.
Benson, Marion T., 501 Century Bldg., Atlanta, Ga. 4, 5.
Bergener, G. J., Physicians' Bldg., San Francisco. T.
Berlin, Lewis, 420 E. Freemason St., Norfolk, Va. 4.
Bernardy, Henry L., 321 S. 11th St., Philadelphia. 2.
Bill, Arthur H., 310 The Osborn Bldg., Cleveland. 4.
Black, Carl E., 349 E. State St., Jacksonville, Ill. T.
Black, Wm. T., 620 Exchange Bldg. Memphis, Tenn. T.
Bland, P. B., 1621 Spruce St., Philadelphia. 9, 1, 2, 4.
Blazejewski, S. W., 103 N. Jordan St., Shenandoah, Pa. 4.
Blesh, A. L. 606-610 State Nat. Bk. Bldg., Oklahoma City. T.
Block, Frank Benton, 1503 Girard Ave., Philadelphia. 4.
Boice, J. Morton, 4020 Spruce St., Philadelphia. 4.
Boldt, Herman J., 39 E. 61st St., New York City. 6, 7, 8, 9, 0, 2, 4.
Bonifield, C. L., 1763 E. McMillan Ave., Avondale, Cincinnati. 4, 5, 6, 7, 8, 2, 4.
Booth, J. C., Main St., Lebanon, Ore. 5.
Bourland, J. W., 3505 Oak Lawn Ave., Dallas, Texas. 3.
Bovée, J. Wesley, The Rochambeau, Washington, D. C. 4, 6, 7, 9, 2, 4.
Bowen, W. Sinclair, 1339 Connecticut Ave., Washington, D. C. 4
Bowers, Chas. E., Beacon Bldg., Wichita, Kan. T.
Bowers, L. G., 141 W. 4th St., Dayton, Ohio. 8, 9, 1, 5.
Bowman, John W., Lemoyne, Pa. 2.
Bowser, W. F., Elberon, Iowa. T.
Boxer, Henry, Empire Bldg., Birmingham, Ala. 3.
Boyd, D. H., 2345 Perrysville St., Pittsburgh. 0, 4.
Boyd, G. M., 1909 Spruce St., Philadelphia. 4, 6, 9, 2, 4.

Boys, C. E., 1404 Portage St., Kalamazoo, Mich. 8, 3.
Boysen, eter, Pelican Rapids, Minn. P
Bozenhardt, William F., 50 Forest Ave., Brooklyn. 2.
Braasch, W. F., Rochester, Minn. 1.
Brack, Chas. Emil, 500 E. 20th St., Baltimore. 2.
Branch, J. R. B., 317 Orange St., Macon, Ga. T.
Branson, L. H, 103 S. Clinton St., Iowa City, Ia. 5, 6, 7, 8, 1, 3, 4.
Branton, B. J., Willmar, Minn. 3.
Bratrud, Theodore, Warren, Minn. T.
Braunwarth, Emma L., 112 E. 2d St., Muscatine, Iowa. 6, 1.
Bray, Charles W., 81 Free St., Portland, Maine. T.
Breck, Samuel, 238 Newbury St., Boston. T.
Brecker, N. Francis, 2347 St. Albans St., Philadelphia. 4.
Breitstein, L. I., 516 Sutter Bldg., San Francisco. 5.
Bresee, Paul, 909 Los Angeles Invest. Bldg., 8th and Broadway, Los Angeles. 1.
Breyer, John H., 1516 N. Los Robles St., Pasadena, Calif. 5.
Brickell, J. B., Americus, Kan. 1.
Brickner, Samuel N., Saranac Lake, N. Y. 2.
Briggs, H. 1026 Jackson St., Wilmington Del. 6, 7, 9, 2.
Brinkman, J. E., 528 Commercial St., Waterloo, Iowa. 3.
Broad, George B., 606 E. Genesee St., Syracuse. 2.
Broadrup, G. L., 203 Virginia Ave., Cumberland, Md. 6, 9, 1, 2, 4.
Brockman, D. C., Ottumwa, Iowa. T.
Broun, LeRoy, 148 W. 77th St., New York City. 2, 4.
Brown, Adelaide, 45 16th Ave., San Francisco. 3.
Brown, Columbus, Herrin, Ill. 0.
Brown, Ellen E., 714 Madison St., Chester, Pa. 4.
Brown, E. L., 608 Livingston Bldg., Bloomington, Ill. 4.
Brown, Ewing, 3405 Farnam St., Omaha, Neb. 3.
Brown, Wm. M., 1776 East Ave., Rochester, N. Y. 2.
Brownsill, Edith S., 2704 College Ave., Berkeley, Calif. 5.
Bryson, Chas. W., 801 City Nat. Bk. Bldg., Los Angeles. 1.
Bullard, R. T., 1241 W. 8th St., Los Angeles. 5, 9, 0, 1, 2, 5.
Bunting, P. D., 1060 E. Jersey St., Elizabeth, N. J. 9, 4.
Burch, L. E., Eve Bldg., Nashville, Tenn. 6, 9, 4.
Burckhardt, Louis, 620 Hume-Mansur Bldg., Indianapolis. 3.
Burke, E. W., Masonic Temple, Redlands, Calif. 4.
Burkhardt, E. D., Del Agua, Colo. 3.
Burkhardt, C. F., Effingham, Ill. 0.
Burnam, Curtis F., 1418 Eutaw Pl., Baltimore. 2, 4, 5.
Burns, T. M., 640 Metropolitan Bldg., Denver. 0, 1, 2, 4.

Buteau, S. H., 1307 Broadway, Oakland, Calif. 5.

Butz, R. E., 103 E. Market St., York, Pa. 4, 6, 1, 2.

Cabot, Hugh, 87 Marlboro St., Boston. T.

Cadwallader, I. H., 919 Taylor Ave., St. Louis. T.

Cain, C. L., Elmwood, Wis. 3.

Calbreath, C. B., Hastings, Neb. T.

Calkins, F. R., 4 Cleveland Bldg., Watertown, N. Y. T.

Campbell, Harry M., 1206 Market St., Parkersburg, W. Va. 1.

Carpenter, H. L., Richmond, Calif. 5.

Carpenter, Frank B., 3966 Washington St., San Francisco. 1.

Carstens, J. H., 1447-55 David Whitney Bldg., Detroit. 4, 5, 6, 7, 9, 0, 2, 3, 4.

Cates, A. B., 2824 Park Ave., Minneapolis. 3.

Cathcart, Robert S., 55 Hasell St., Charleston, S. C. T.

Catlin, S. R., 204 Masonic Temple, Rockford, Ill. T.

Chace, Archibald E., 76 Broadway, Tarrytown, N. Y. 4.

Chadbourn, A. G., Heron Lake, Minn. 3.

Chalfant, Sidney A., 5713 Rippey St., Pittsburgh. 0, 2.

Chandler, S., 1935 Spruce St., Philadelphia. 4, 6, 7, 9, 2, 4.

Chapman, W. E., Litchfield, Minn. 3.

Chard, Marie L., 616 Madison Ave., New York City. 9, 2, 3, 4.

Chatterton, A. S., Peterson, Ia. 3.

Clark, Chester H., 4301 Superior St., Duluth, Minn. 3.

Clark, E. S., Sumas, Wash. T.

Clark, J. A., 30 N. Michigan Blvd., Chicago. 1.

Clark, John G., 2017 a nut St., Philadelphia. 4, 6, 9W0J 2, 4.

Clark, S. M. D., 1619 Arabella St., New Orleans, La. 6, 9, 1, 2, 3, 5.

Clarke, Austin F., Bk. of Sav. Bldg., Oakland, Calif. 5.

Clarke, Genevieve, 825 Mass. Ave., Cambridge, Mass. 5.

Clarke, Wm. T., 1777 W. Jefferson St., Los Angeles. 1.

Clarkson, W. H., Manhattan, Kan. 1.

Clawson, Marcus L., 420 Park Ave., Plainfield, N. J. 2.

Clegg, J. T., Siloam Springs, Ark. 0, 1.

Coates, Benj. O., 221 North Euclid Ave., Pasadena, Cal. 1.

Cobb, W. F., Lyle, Minn. 3.

Coe, Henry C., 8 W. 76th St., New York City. 2.

Coffey, R. C., 789 Glisem St., Portland, Ore. T.

Coffey, Titian, 926 Marsh-Strong Bldg., Los Angeles. 1.

Cogill, Lida Stewart, 1831 Chestnut St., Philadelphia. 2, 4.

Cohen, Bernard, 568 Lafayette Ave., Buffalo. T.

Cole, C. Grenes, 1109 Maison Blanche Bldg., New Orleans. 4.

Coles, Stricker, 2103 Walnut St., Philadelphia. 4, 9, 2, 4.

Colgan, Jas. F. E., 1022 N. 5th St., Philadelphia. 4.

Collins, Clifford Bldg., Peoria, T.

Collins, J. L., Sheffield, Iowa. 3.

Comfort, Clifford V. C., 512 Mercantile Bldg., Rochester, N. Y. 2.

Commiskey, Leo J. J., 189 6th Ave., Brooklyn. 2.

Comstock, George F., 540 Broadway, Saratoga Springs, N. Y. T.

Conaway, W. P., 1723 Pacific Ave., Atlantic City, N. J. 4, 9, 2, 3, 4.

Congdon, Charles E., 859 Humboldt St., Buffalo. 2.

Conner, A. L., 7056 Main St., Philadelphia. 7, 2.

Conrad, S. Alvin, Leetonia, Ohio. 4, 5.

Conrad, Thos. K., Chevy Chase, Md. 4.

Conway, H. P., Spring Valley, Wis. 3.

Coon, W. F., Caney, Kan. 3.

Cootes, Thos. G., 1413 Lombard St., Philadelphia. 4.

Cordier, A. H., 510 Commerce Bldg., Kansas City, Mo. T.

Corwin, R. W., Minnequa Hosp., Pueblo, Colo. T.

Cory, W. M., Waterville, Minn. 3.

Cosgrave, Millicent, 350 Post St., San Francisco. 1.

Councilman, W. T., 78 Bay State Road, Boston. T.

Cousins, Wm. L., 231 Woodfords St., Portland, Maine. 4.

Coventry, W. A., 1921 E. 3d St., Duluth, Minn. 4.

Cowles, J. E., 524 Mer. Nat. Bank Bldg., Los Angeles. 1, 5.

Cox, Thos. J., 701 Eye St., Sacramento, Calif. T.

Craig, N. S., Jennings, La. 8, 3.

Creamer, Michael S., 501 Homer Laughlin Blk., Los Angeles. 1.

Crotty, Nora, 909 Union Central Bldg., Cincinnati. 2.

Crowley, Daniel F., 208 Flynn Bldg., Des Moines, Iowa. 3.

Culbertson, Emma B., 33 Newbury St., Boston. 3.

Cullen, T. S., 20 E. Eager St., Baltimore. 4, 6, 7, 8, 3, 4.

Cunningham, S. P., 116 West Woodlawn Ave., San Antonio, Texas. T.

Daniels, C. D., 2267 N. 18th St., Philadelphia. 4.

Dannreuther, Walter T., 2030 Broadway, New York City. 2, 4.

Darling, Chas. B., 50 Townsend St., Boston. 6, 1.

Darnall, W. E., 1704 Pacific Ave., Atlantic City, N. J. 6, 9, 2, 4.

Darnell, C. F., Llano, Texas. T.

Davenport, James Henry, 210 Benefit St., Providence. 2.

Davidson, H. A., 418 Atherton Bldg., Louisville, Ky. 4.

Davies, Wm. Rowland, 221 S. Main Ave., Scranton, Pa. 3, 4.

Davis, Albert B., 511 Cooper St., Camden, N. J. 2, 4.

Davis, Asa Barnes, 42 E. 35th St., New York City. 4.
Davis, B. B., Bee Bldg., Omaha, T.
Davis, Carl H., 25 E. Washington St., Chicago. 5.
Davis, E. C., 25 E. Linden St., Atlanta, Ga. 0, 2, 3, 4, 5.
Davis, Edward P., 250 S. 21st St., Philadelphia. 6, 7, 2, 4.
Davis, Ella M., 188 Chestnut St., Holyoke, Mass. 9, 4.
Davis, J. C., 19 Cumberland St., Rochester, N. Y. 4 9, 2.
Davis, John D. S., 2031 G Ave., Birmingham, Ala. 6, 7, 0, 2.
Davis, W. J., 229 Barney St., Wilkes-Barre, Pa. 2.
Davison, Robert E., 8152 Jenkins Arcade Bldg., Pittsburgh. T.
Deaver, John B., 1634 Walnut St., Philadelphia. 4.
Delaney, Chas. W., 1320 9th St., Altoona, Pa. T.
DeLee, J. B., 5028 Ellis Ave., Chicago. 8, 2, 3, 4, 5.
Denney, Jos. C., Clyde Park, Mont. 3.
Dennis, Mary E., 1217 Trenton St., Los Angeles. 1.
DeVenney, J. C., 1115 N. 2d St., Harrisburg, Pa. 2.
Dickinson, Robert L., 168 Clinton St., Brooklyn. 2, 4.
Diez, M. Luise, 5733 Spruce St., Philadelphia. 2.
Dilliard, Benjamin F., Central St., East Bangor, Pa. 2.
Disen, Chas. F., 2600 E. 22d St., Minneapolis. 3.
Ditchburn, D. T., Arnot, Pa. 5.
Dodds, Robt., 3946 Cottage Grove Ave., Chicago. 4.
Dodge, Roy A., 446 Brandeis Bldg., Omaha, Neb. 3.
Donaldson, Harry J., 106 E. 4th St., Williamsport, Pa. 4.
Donoghue, Francis D., 864 Beacon St., Boston. 5, 6, 7, 9, 2.
Dowdall, Richard J., 6 Raymond Ave., San Francisco. 5
Dowling, Oscar, Commercial Nat. Bk. Bldg., Shreveport, La. T.
Downs, A. J., 303 Johnson Blk., Los Angeles. 0, 1, 5.
Downs, R. N., Jr., 6008 Greene St., Philadelphia. 4.
Dowman, Chas. E., Jr., 1618 Candler Bldg., Atlanta, Ga. 4.
Doyle, O. B., Box 913, Fresno, Cal. 1, 5.
Dozier, Linwood, 221 Elks Bldg., Stockton, Calif. 5.
Drayer, L. P., Fort Wayne, Ind. T.
Du Bose, F. G., Selma, Ala. 4.
Duffield, William, Auditorium Bldg., Los Angeles. 5.
Duffy, Ralph, Plant City, Fla. T.
Dugdale, R. B., 127 S. Lafayette St., South Bend, Ind. 1.
Dukes, Charles A., Central Bk. Bldg., Oakland, Calif. 5.
Duncan, H. A., 2721 W. Lehigh Ave., Philadelphia. 9, 2.
Dunn, J. E., Stratford, S. Dak. 3.
Dunshee, J. D., Keystone, Iowa. T.

Dunsmoor, F. A., 100 Andrews Bldg., Minneapolis. T.
Dunsmoor, John M., 506 Stimson Bldg., Los Angeles. 1.
Dunsmoor, Nannie C., 1105 Garland Bldg., Los Angeles. 1, 5.
Durrie, Anna B., % Colo. Sanit., Boulder, Colo. 1.
Dwire, Francis B., Gardena, Calif. 1.
Earle, C. B., Main and North Sts., Greenville, S. C. T.
Eastland, Doyle L., 1003 Amicable Bldg., Waco, Texas. T.
Eastman, T. B., 308 Pennway Bldg., Indianapolis. 5, 8, 3.
Eaton, Alvin R., Jr., 1157 E. Jersey St., Elizabeth, N. J. 2.
Echols, C. M., 800 Majestic Bldg., Milwaukee, Wis. 2, 3, 4.
Edwards, Thos. C., 224½ Main St., Salinas, Cal. 1.
Elkin, W. S., 1029 Candler Bldg., Atlanta, Ga. 2.
Ellis, Wm. Clyde, 115 W. Monroe St., Phoenix, Ariz. 1.
Elsey, J. R., Glenwood, Minn. 3.
English, C. H., Fort Wayne, Ind. 8, 2.
Equi, Marie D., Central Bldg., Portland, Ore. 4.
Erck, Theo. A., 251 S. 13th St., Philadelphia. 2.
Eschleman, L. H., 2923 S. Washington St., Marion, Ind. 3.
Eskridge, Belle C., 412 Temple Bldg., Houston, Tex. 4.
Evans, C. M., Clifford, Ill. 4.
Ewer, Edward N., 176 Santa Rosa Ave., Oakland, Calif. 5, 1, 5.
Fair, H. D., 103 Vatel Bldg., Muncie, Ind. 4.
Fair, Robert P., 481 Beacon St., Boston. 2.
Fairbanks, C., 24 Main St., St. Johnsbury, Vt. 4.
Fairchild, F. D., 4521 Central Ave., Los Angeles. 1.
Faisau, W. F., 45 Greenwood Ave., Jersey City, N. J. 5.
Falls, F. H., 2800 Washington Blvd., Chicago. 4.
Farrar, Lillian K. P., 40 W. 96th St., New York City. 4.
Favill, H. B., 122 S. Michigan Ave., Chicago. T.
Fay, G. H., Auburn, Calif. 5.
Feeley, Matilda A., 1700 Sutter St., San Francisco. 1.
Feidt, Wilson Wellington, 1028 Andrus Bldg., Minneapolis. 3.
Fifield, Emily W., 431 Syndicate Blk., Minneapolis. 3.
Findley, Palmer, 3602 Lincoln Blvd., Omaha. 1, 2.
Finley, C. S., 104 ast 40th St., New York City. 2E3.
Fisher, John M., 222 S. 15th St., Philadelphia. 6, 7, 9, 4.
Fisher, W. H., 4163 Colton Bldg., Toledo, Ohio. 8, .
Fithian, J. W., 608 Broadway, Camden, N. J. 6, 9, 2, 4.
Fitzgerald, William W., Box 113, Stockton, Calif. 5.
Flagg, Chas. E. B., 1409 Columbia St., Vancouver, Wash. T.

Hannah, Calvin R., 512 S. W. Life Bldg., Dallas, Tex. 4.

Hanson, Geo. C., 205-6 Cobb Bldg., Seattle, Wash. 3.

Harbert, G. E., Beverly, N. J. 2, 4.

Hare, Chas. B., Bk. of San Jose Bldg., San Jose, Calif. 5.

Harman, Wm. J., 1162 E. State St., Trenton, N. J. 2.

Harris, Philander A., 453 Park Ave., Paterson, N. J. 6, 7, 9, 3, 4.

Harris, M. L., 25 E. Washington St., Chicago. T.

Harry, Charles R., 54 Physicians' Bldg., Stockton, Calif. T.

Hart, Frank E., 1200 S. Market St., Canton, Ohio. T.

Hart, Robt. S., Turton, S. D. 3.

Harter, Isaac F., Stronghurst, Ill. 1.

Hartley, Harriet L., 1534 N. 15th St., Philadelphia. 4.

Hartman, John V., Findlay, Ohio. 3.

Hartwell, D. D., Marion, Ill. 3.

Hartz, Harry J., 1002 Jackson St., Philadelphia. 4.

Harvey, E. M., Media, Pa. 9, 2.

Harvey, E. H., 20 N. Florida Ave., Atlantic City, N. J. 2.

Hawkes, E. W. Z., 14 Fulton St., Newark, N. J. T.

Hayd, Herman E., 493 Delaware Ave., Buffalo. 4.

Hayden, A. M., Evansville, Ind. 3, 4.

Hayes, Nellie S., 306 Ferguson Bldg., Los Angeles. 1, 5.

Heaney, N. Sproat, 5548 Woodlawn Ave., Chicago. 3.

Heflin, Wyatt, Birmingham, Ala. 4.

Heimark, A. J., Finley, N. D. 3.

Heineberg, Alfred, 1642 Pine St., Philadelphia. 9, 2.

Heinecke, Geo. B., 5634 Georgia Ave. N.W., Washington, D. C. 9, 2.

Heisz, Emily J., 345 E. Ocean Ave., Long Beach, Calif. 1, 5.

Heller, Jacob, 1199 eastern Parkway, New York City. 2, 4.

Helm, W. B., Rockford, Ill. T.

Helms, John S., American Nat. Bk. Bldg., Tampa, Fla. T.

Hendon, George A., Highland and Baxter Aves., Louisville, Ky. T.

Henry, Clifford E., 715 Donaldson Bldg., Minneapolis. 3.

Henry, E. C., 610 Brandeis Theater Bldg., Omaha. T.

Henry, W. O., 614 Brandeis Theater Bldg., Omaha, Neb. 2, 3.

Hensel, Chas. N., 223 Moore Bldg., St. Paul. 3.

Herrman, Max F., 3703 Old York Rd., Philadelphia. 4.

Hertzler, Arthur E., Halsted, Kan. 1, 4.

Herzog, Geo. K., 133 Geary St., San Francisco. 1, 5.

Hewitt, Sophie B. K., 135 Stockton St., San Francisco. 5.

Higgins, C. W., 2 George St., Providence, R. I. 4, 6, 7, 9, 2.

Highsmith, J. F., Fayettesville, N. C. T.

Hilkowich, A. M., 1057 Hoe Ave., Bronx, New York City. 2.

Hill, Howard, 1010 Rialto Bldg., Kansas City, Mo. T.

Hill, W. B., 507 39th St., Milwaukee, Wis. 9, 2.

Hipke, G. A., 3021 Cedar St., Milwaukee, Wis. 8, 10.

Hirschfield, Adolph, 1017 Washington Ave., N., Minneapolis. 3.

Hirschfield, M. S., New Jersey Bldg., Duluth, Minn. 3.

Hobbs, Alice L., 5828 E. Washington St., Indianapolis. 8, 1.

Hoffman, C. S., Keyser, W. Va. 0, 2.

Hoffmann, Chas. von, 2669 California St., San Francisco. 1, 5.

Hoffman, Lawrence H., 530 Butler Bldg., San Francisco. 5.

Hoffman, R. C., Deming, N. M. T.

Hohf, S. M., 115 West 3d St., Yankton, S. D. T.

Holden, Frederick C., 198 Lincoln Pl., Brooklyn. 4.

Holmes, Rudolph W., 33 E. Elm St., Chicago. 4, 8, 3.

Holmes, Will H., 352 Pomona Invest Bldg., Pomona, Calif. 5.

Hollister, J. C., 302 Dodsworth Bldg., Pasadena, Calif. 1.

Holsti, Osten, Electric Bldg., Aberdeen, Wash. 5.

Hood, C. S., Ferndale, Wash. 5.

Horigan, J. A., 1107 E. 53rd St., Kansas City, Mo. 5.

Hornibrook, E., Cherokee, Iowa. 1.

Horsley, J. Shelton, 617 W. Grace St., Richmond, Va. 3.

Houck, Mary P., 816 Main St., La Crosse, Wis. 3.

Howard, A. Philo, 431 Kress Bldg., Houston, Texas. T.

Hromadka, A. B., Sawtelle, Calif. 1.

Hubert, R. I., 853 Iglehart Ave., St. Paul. 3.

Hudston, Ranulph, Metropolitan Bldg., Denver. 5.

Huggins, R. R., 1018 Westinghouse Bldg., Pittsburgh. 0, 2, 4.

Humiston, Wm. H., 536 Rose Bldg., Cleveland. 4.

H   Tornius Blk.,

H

H

H

Hupp, Frank LeMoyne, 61 14th St., Wheeling, W. Va. T.

Hutchins, H. T., 522 Commonwealth Ave., Boston. 2.

Ill, Edgar A., 192 Clinton Ave., Newark, N. J. 4.

Ill, Edw. J., 1002 Broad St., Newark, N. J. 9, 2, 4.

Ingraham, Clarence B., Jr., 668 Metropolitan Bldg., Denver. 1.

Ireland, Milton S., 23 S. California St., Atlantic City, N. J. 4.

Ireland, R. Lindsey, 600 The Atherton Bldg., Louisville, Ky. T.

Irwin, John R., 401 N. Tryon St., Charlotte, N. C. 1.

Lindahl, John, 1434 Glenarm, Denver. 5.
Linder, Wm., 889 St. Marks Ave., Brooklyn. T.
Lindley, Walter, 1414 S. Hope St., Los Angeles. 5, 1.
Lindsay, Kate, Sanitarium, Boulder, Colo. 3.
Linklater, Eugene R., 233 W. Utica St., Buffalo. 3.
Lipes, H. Judson, 178 Washington Ave., Albany, N. Y. T.
Littig, Lawrence W., Putnam Bldg., Davenport, Iowa. T.
Litzenberg, J. C., 3137 Park Ave., Minneapolis. 6, 8, 2, 3, 5.
Livingston, W. R., 426 B St., Oxnard, Calif. 5.
Lockrey, Sarah H., 1520 Vine St., Philadelphia. 4, 8, 9, 2.
Long, John Wesley, 115 Church St., Greensboro, N. C. 4.
Long, Wm. H., 4657 Lancaster Ave., Philadelphia. 4.
Longaker, Daniel, 344 N. 5th St., Philadelphia. 4.
Longenecker, C. B., 3416 arin St., Philadelphia. 4, 6, 9, 2 4. g
Longyear, H. W., 708-710 Shurley Bldg., Detroit. T.
Loomis, E. E., Janesville, Wis. 6, 1.
Looney, Robt. N., Prescott, Ariz. 1.
Loper, A. N., Box 121, Dinuba, Calif. T.
Loranger, Philip J., 383 Canton Ave., Detroit. 3.
Lorentz, Robert, 2227 Fulton St., San Francisco. 5.
Losee, J. R., 307 2d Ave., New York City. 4, 5.
Loughridge, Sherman, Grants Pass, Ore. 5.
Luburg, L. F., 1822 irar Ave., Philadelphia. 9, 2, 4G d
Luther, F. M., 610 W. 113th St., New York City. 2.
Lutz, F. J., 3337 Lafayette Ave., St. Louis, Mo. T.
Lyman, C. B., 416 Metropolitan Bldg., Denver.
Lyman, J. V. R.T Ingram Bldg., Eau Claire, Wis. T.
Lyons, J. A., 6848 Anthony Ave., Chicago. 8, 3.
MacCarroll, D. R., 2503 S. Broad St., Philadelphia. 2, 4.
MacEvitt, John C., 407 Clinton St., Brooklyn. 1, 2, 3, 5.
MacKellar, Jas., 71 N. Church St., Hazleton, Pa. 4.
MacKenzie, John R., Carington, N. D. 3.
Mackenzie, K. A. J., 908 Corbett Bldg., Portland, Ore. T.
Magee, M. D'Arcy, 1623 Connecticut Ave., Washington, D. C. 3.
Magee, W. G., Granite Blk., Watertown, S. D. 3.
Magie, W. H., 1401 E. Superior St., Duluth, Minn. T.
Magill, Wm. H., 221 Thayer St., Providence, R. I. 2.
Mahoney, S. A., 630 Dwight St., Holyoke, Mass. T.

Maier, F. Hurst, 1900 Chestnut St., Philadelphia. 4.
Maison, Robert S., Chester, Pa. 2.
Mallett, G. H., 244 W. 73d St., New York City. 9, 2.
Malone, W. F., 324 Madison St., Milwaukee. T.
Mangan, P. J., Winnemucca, Nev. 5.
Manion, Katherine C., Corbett Bldg., Portland, Ore. 5.
Mann, Bernard, 107 N. 60th St., Philadelphia. 4.
Manton, W. P., 32 W. Adams Ave., Detroit. 4, 5, 6, 7, 8, 9, 0, 2.
March, E. J., 322 S. Cleveland Ave., Canton, Ohio. 4, 9, 0, 1, 2, 3, 4.
arcy, Henry O., 180 Commonwealth Ave., Boston. 4, 6, 7, 8, 9, 0, 2, 3, 4, 5.
Markoe, Jas. W., 20 W. 50th St., New York City. 2, 3.
Marshall, Clara, 258 S. 16th St., Philadelphia. 0, 1.
artin, E. D., 1428 Josephine St., New Orleans. T.
M   Ave.,
M   dway,
M   Ave.,
                     J. T.
16 Pacific Ave.,
                     J. T.
n, Sanit., 1823
iladelphia. 4, 6,
822 Hudson St.,
9, 2, 4.
Memphis Trust
Tenn. 4.
408 Donaldson
3.
Central Ave.,
3.
M   17 Brockman
1.
M   Ponce, P. R.
McAllister, Anna M., 3503 Baring St., Philadelphia. 4.
McCabe, W. M., City Hosp., Nashville, Tenn. 3.
McCannel, A. J., Minot, N. D. 3.
McCarty, T. L., Dodge City, Kan. 3.
McCay, Robt. Burns, 228 Chestnut St., Sunbury, Pa. 4.
McChord, Robert C., Lebanon, Ky. T.
McCown, O. S., Memphis Trust Bldg., Memphis, Tenn. T.
McCoy, John C., 292 Broadway, Paterson, N. J. T.
McCoy, John H., Beattie, Kan. 3.
McCracken, R. W., Union Grove, Wis. 8, 3.
McCullough, A. H., 78 W. Park Ave., Mansfield, Ohio. 3.
McDaniel, E. B., 703 Electric Bldg., Portland, Ore. T.
McDavitt, Thomas, Lowry Bldg., St. Paul. T.
                         n St.,
                         bard

McEwen, Mary G., 1703 Chicago Ave., Evanston, Ill. 0, 3.

McGlinn, John A., 113 S. 20th St., Philadelphia. 9, 2.

McKee, E. S., 2132 Sinton Ave., Cincinnati. 5, 6, 7, 8, 0, 5.

McKenney, D. C., 1250 Main St., Buffalo. 9, 3.

McLaren, J. L., Title Insurance Bldg., Los Angeles. 4, 5.

McMahon, J. P., 406 Cudahy Apts., Milwaukee, Wis. 3.

McMullen, B. H., 210 Cass St., Cadillac, Mich. 4.

McMurtry, L. S., 5 Ormsby Pl., Louisville, Ky. 4, 5, 6, 7, 8, 0, 2, 3, 4.

McNamara, Sylvester J., 369 Union St., Brooklyn. 4.

McNeil, H. S., Exchange Bldg., Los Angeles. 5.

McNeile, Lyle G., 626 Marsh-Strong Bldg., Los Angeles. 1, 5.

McNeile, Olga, Marsh Strong Bldg., Los Angeles. 5.

McNutt, Sarah J., 265 Lexington Ave., New York City. 9, 0, 2.

McNutt, W. F., Butler Bldg., San Francisco. 5.

McPherson, Ross, 20 W. 50th St., New York City. 8, 9, 0, 2, 3.

McReynolds, R. P., B. F. Coulter Bldg., Los Angeles. 4, 5.

McSweeney, P. E., 46 N. Champlain St., Burlington, Vt. 4.

McVea, C., Roumain Bldg., Baton Rouge, La. T.

Meads, Albert M., 2216 College Ave., Berkeley, Calif. 5.

Meanes, L. L., 302 Securities Bldg., Des Moines, Iowa. 2.

Megrail, W. P., Penn and Zane St., Wheeling, W. Va. 4.

Meigs, J. V., 160 Merrimack, Lowell, Mass. T.

Meirerding, Wm. A., Springfield, Minn. 3.

Mellby, O. F., Thief River Falls, Minn. 3.

Melvin, J. Tracy, Porterville, Calif. 1.

Mendenhall, T. E., 432 Lincoln St., Johnstown, Pa. 4.

Mensel, Harry H., 65 Main St., Oshkosh, Wis. 3.

Mercer, Clarence, Gross Bldg., Eureka, Calif. 5.

Mertens, J. J., Gettysburg, S. D. T.

Messinger, M. P., Oakfield, N. Y. 3.

Metcalf, Wm. F., 1045 D. Whitney Bldg., Detroit. T.

Meyers, Elmer L., 17 W. South St., Wilkes-Barre, Pa. 2.

Michaux, Stuart, 926 West Franklin St., Richmond, Va. 2.

Miller, C. Jeff, 1638 Joseph St., New Orleans. 6, 7, 8, 9, 0, 1, 2, 4.

Miller, Harold A., 617 Pittsburgh Life Bldg., Pittsburgh. 9, 2, 4.

Miller, John D., Norfolk Bldg., Cincinnati. 4.

Miller, Mary T., 313 N. 33d St., Philadelphia. 2, 4.

Miller, S. M., Box 544, Knoxville, Tenn. 9, 1, 4.

Miller, Theo., 1826 Euclid Ave., Cleveland. 4.

Miller, V. A., Lake Arthur, La. 8, 3.

Miller, W. E., Columbus, Ill. 8, 1.

Mills, Henry M., 192A 6th Ave., Brooklyn. 6, 7, 9, 2.

Mills, W. P., Missoula, Mont. T.

Milton, J. L., 3020 Telegraph Ave., Oakland, Calif. T.

Mitchell, John H., 305 N. 16th St., Mt. Vernon, Ill. 0, 4.

Mitchell, Ralph S., Grand Meadow, Minn. 3.

Mitchell, Robert L., 2112 Maryland Ave., Baltimore. 9, 4.

Mock, Harry E., 7409 Sheridan Rd., Chicago. 3.

Molz, Chas., Murphysboro, Ill. 4.

Montgomery, E. E., 1426 Spruce St., Philadelphia. 4, 5, 6, 7, 8, 9, 0, 1, 2, 3, 4, 5.

Montgomery, F. H., 478 W. Broadway, Danville, Ky. 3.

Moore, Chester B., 291 Geary St., San Francisco. 5.

Moore, James S., Medical Bldg., Portland, Ore. 1.

Moore, M. L., 340 S. Kinsley Drive, Los Angeles. 1.

Moore, W. G., 177 Port St., San Francisco. 5.

Moore, Will H., Sykeston, N. D. 3.

Moots, Charles W., The Nicholas, Toledo, Ohio. T.

Moran, John F., 2420 Penn. Ave., Washington, D. C. 4.

Morehouse, G. G., Hotel Owatonna, Owatonna, Minn. 3.

Moriarta, D. C., 511 Broadway, Saratoga, N. Y. T.

Morris, Charles A., Bower Bldg., Bakersfield, Calif. 5.

Morris, E. J., 488 9th St., Brooklyn. 2, 4.

Morris, L. C., 1203 m ire Bldg., Birmingham, Ala. Æ4p

Morris, Margaret M., 608 Hollingsworth Bldg., Los Angeles. 1.

Morrison, John B., 97 Halsey St., Newark, N. J. 4.

Morrison, N. D., 3d St., San Mateo, Calif. 1.

Morse, Arthur H., University Hosp., San Francisco. 5.

Morse, W. B., Holman Bldg., Salem, Ore. T.

Mortensen, Wm. S., Palms, Calif. 1.

Morton, Ada S. C., 901 Butler Bldg., San Francisco. 3.

Morton, Rosalie S., Hotel Lenori, 63d and Madison Ave., New York City. 4.

Mosher, Clelia D., 1094 Emerson St., Palo Alto, Calif. 4.

Mount, Walter B., 21 Plymouth St., Montclair, N. J. 4.

Moynihan, T. J., 2391½ University Ave., St. Paul. T.

Mueller, Geo., 2024 Pierce Ave., Chicago. T.

Munger, I. C., Cozad, Neb. 5

Munter, Leo, 515 Hewes Bldg., San Francisco. 1, 5.

Murdoch, H. G., Taylor's Falls, Minn. 3.

Murphy, Wm. B., 2652 Bloomington Ave., Minneapolis. 3.

Murray, Grace P., 50 W. 45th St., New York City. 2.

Murray, Janet, 14 Mynderse St., Schenectady, N. Y. 1.

Muse, B. P., 1039 Edmondson Ave., Baltimore. 4.

Naegeli, Frank, Manhattan Bldg., Fergus Falls, Minn. 3.

Nakabayashi, M., 1811 Pine St., San Francisco. 5.

Nash, A. B., 10 S. 13th St., Newark, N. J. 2.

Neer, William, 245 Broadway, Paterson, N. J. T.

Neff, G. R., Farmington, Iowa. 0, 1.

Newman, Henry P., 1560 8th St., San Diego, Calif. 4, 6, 0, 1, 2, 5.

Newton, John C., 291 Geary St., San Francisco. 1, 5.

Ney, K. Winfield, Madisonville, La. T.

Nieder, Chas. F., 140 Genesee St., Geneva, N. Y. 4.

Nielson, A. F. O., Oakley, Idaho. 3.

Nihiser, Winton M., 128 E. Antietam St., Hagerstown, Md. 4.

Noble, Mary Riggs, 706 N. Nevada Ave., Colorado Springs, Colo. 5.

Noble, Thos. B., 720 Newton Claypool Bldg., Indianapolis. 2.

Norris, R. C., 500 N. 20th St., Philadelphia. 4, 9, 2.

Novak, Emil, 26 E. Preston St., Baltimore, Md. 9, 0, 2, 4.

Nye, H. W., Osborne, Kan. 3.

Oates, T. K., cor. Maple and Burke Sts., Martinsburg, W. Va. T.

O'Connor, T. H., Clements 453, San Francisco. T.

Ogden, B. H., 546 Holly Ave., St. Paul. 3.

Ogilvie, H. H., 541 Moore Bldg., San Antonio, Texas. T.

Old, Wm. L., 307 Taylor Bldg., Norfolk, Va. T.

Oppegaard, M. O., New London, Minn. 3.

Orella, F. R., 323 Geary St., San Francisco. 5.

Osborn, Geo. R., 805 Jefferson Ave., La Porte, Ind. 2, 4.

Osborne, Daniel E., St. Helena, Calif. 5.

Outerbridge, Geo. W., 2040 Chestnut St., Philadelphia. 4.

Overton, John, % Dr. Wagner, Palace Bldg., Tulsa, Okla. 3.

Page, Addison C., 210 Equitable Bldg., Des Moines, Iowa. 3.

Palmer, Carolina B., 2401 Sacramento St., San Francisco. 5.

Palmer, Sarah E., 483 Beacon St., Boston. 4.

Pampel, B. L., Livingston, Mont. 3.

Pancoast, Henry K., Box 203, Bala, Pa. 4.

Pantzer, H. O., 717 Woodruff Pl., Indianapolis. 4, 5, 6, 7, 8, 9, 0, 2, 4, 5.

Parham, F. W., 1429 Seventh St., New Orleans. T.

Park, Frederick S., 4106 Girard Ave., Philadelphia. 4.

Parke, Wm. E., 1739 N. 17th St., Philadelphia. 4, 9, 2.

Parker, L. Maud, Lumber Exchange, Seattle, Wash. 4, 5.

Parmenter, Geo. H., 106 E. State St., Montpelier, Vt. 3.

Parry, Angenette, 749 Madison Ave., New York City. 2, 5.

Parsonnet, Victor, 124 W. Kinney St., Newark, N. J. 2, 4.

Parsons, H. J., Mansfield, La. T.

Pascoe, M. W., Taft, Calif. 5.

Patterson, Robt. U., U. S. Army, Washington, D. C. 2, 4.

Patton, Chas. L., 628 E. apito St., Springfield, Ill. 0, 3. C 1

Peck, G. S., 408 Stambaugh Bldg., Youngstown, Ohio. T.

Pederson, Reuben M., 801-4 Masonic Temple, Minneapolis. 3.

Peek, Allen, 438 B St., Oxnard, Calif. 5.

Pennington, J. R., 31 N. State St., Chicago. 3, 4, 5.

Perkins, I. B., 132 W. 4th Ave., Denver. T.

Perry, Samuel W., 164 Leasure Ave., New Castle, Pa. 1.

Peters, Lulu H., Melrose Hotel, Los Angeles. 1.

Pfaff, O. G., 338 Newton Claypool Bldg., Indianapolis. 6, 7, 2, 4.

Pfahler, Geo. E., 1321 Spruce St., Philadelphia. 4.

Pfeiffenberger, Mather, Room 5, Lewis Bldg., Alton, Ill. 5.

Phillips, Frederica, 508 Cobb Bldg., Seattle. 5.

211 Goodrich Bldg., z. T.

., 287 Clinton Ave., 6, 7, 9, 1, 2, 3, 4, 5.

310 5th Ave., New York. 3.

Pomeroy, George T., 473 14th St., Oakland, Calif. 5.

Porter, M. C., New England Bldg., Topeka, Kan. T.

Porter, William S., 12th & Broadway, Oakland, Calif. 5.

Potter, I. W., 420 Franklin St., Buffalo. 9, 0, 2.

Potter, Marion Craig, 1487 South Ave., Rochester, N. Y. 9, 2.

Potter, Mary E., 305 Washington Ave., Brooklyn. 5.

Potter, Wm. W., 284 Franklin St., Buffalo. T.

Powell, Cuthbert, Metropolitan Bldg., Denver. T.

Pratt, Chas. A., 60 Orchard St., New Bedford, Mass. T.

Purnell, Caroline M., 132 S. 18th St., Philadelphia. 4, 9, 2, 4.

Pyle, J. L., Chester, W. Va. 4.

Randall, Lillian C., 221 Sherman Ave., New York City. 4.

Rankin, W. H., 151 Hancock St., Brooklyn. 3.

Ratajski, J. E., 16 E. 2d St., Mt. Carmel, Pa. 2, 4.

Raudenbush, J. S., 3633 N. 15th St., Philadelphia. T.

Raymer, H. S., Cedar Rapids, Ia. 3.

Reddan, M. W., 113 W. State St., Trenton, N. J. T.

Reddick, J. T., Paducah, Ky. 6, 7, 1.

Reed, Charles A. L., 180 Union Central Bk. Bldg., Cincinnati. 6, 9, 2, 4.

Reese, Frank D., 16 Tompkins St., Cortland, N. Y. 4.

Reeves, W. R., Salinas, Calif. 5.

Reid, Chas. T., Carona, Kan. T.

Reilly, John P., 215 Elizabeth Ave., Elizabeth, N. J. 2, 4.

Reinle, George G., Macdonough Bldg., Oakland, Calif. T.

Reynolds, Chas. B., 2003 Diamond St., Philadelphia. 9, 2, 4.

Reynolds, E., 321 Dartmouth St., Boston. 6, 7, 3, 5.

Reynolds, H. R., Clinton, Ia. 3.

Reynolds, Robert G., Frazer Bldg., Palo Alto, Calif. 5.

Rhodes, F. A., 914 N. Negley Ave., Pittsburgh. 2.

Rice, E. E., Shawnee, Okla. 8, 1.

Richards, Raymond G., St. David, Ill. 3.

Richardson, Anna G., 483 Beacon St., Boston. 4.

Richardson, Emma M., 581 Stevens St., Camden, N. J. 4, 9, 2, 4.

Richmond, W. W., Clinton, Ky. 5, 1.

Ries, Emil, 30 N. Michigan Ave., Chicago. 0, 3.

Riley, Percy E., Elk Mound, Wis. 3.

Risk, Winthrop A., State Home and School, Providence, R. I. 9, 2.

Ritter, Caleb A., 702 Bryant Bldg., Kansas City, Mo. 0, 2.

Roan, Carl M., 801 Masonic Temple, Minneapolis. 3.

Robb, Hunter, Rose Bldg., Cleveland. 8, 2.

Roberts, W. B., 604 Pillsbury Bldg., Minneapolis. 3, 4.

Robertson, C. H., Holman Bldg., Salem, Ore. T.

Robertson, John B., Cottonwood, Minn. 3.

Robison, Geo. E., Provo Gen. Hosp., Provo, Utah. 5.

Robson, John A., Hall, N. Y. 4.

Rodgers, Chas. L., 700 W. Lake Minneapolis. 3.

Rodi, C. H., Calumet, Mich. T.

Rogers, John T., 209 Lowry Bldg., St. Paul. T.

Rogers, Joseph D., 1400 M St., Washington, D. C. 2, 4.

Rogers, Thos. L., 405 L. B. Bank Bldg., Long Beach, Calif. 1, 5.

Roos, Elias G., 232 Adams Ave., Scranton, Pa. T.

Rongy, A. J., 154 Henry St., New York City. 2, 4.

Rosengren, Chas. J., 218 E. Ferry St., Buffalo. 2, 3, 4, 5.

Rosenthal, Maurice I., Fort Wayne, Ind. T.

Ross, George G., 1721 Spruce St., Philadelphia. T.

Rothenburg, Samuel, 22 W. 7th St., Cincinnati. 1.

Rothrock, J. L., 235 Lowry Arcade, St. Paul. 6, 7, 0, 3.

Rowe, Wm. H., St. James, Minn. 3.

Rubinow, S. M., 602 High St., Newark, N. J. 2.

Rudasill, J. E., Marshall, Va. 2.

Rumford, S. C., 1403 Market St., Wilmington, Del. 2.

Rushmore, Stephen, 520 Beacon St., Boston. 2, 4.

Russ, W. B., 1516 Main Ave., San Antonio, Texas. T.

Russell, Thos. H., Jr., 411 Temple St., New Haven, Conn. 4.

Russell, Wm. W., 1208 Eutaw Pl., Baltimore. 4, 9, 4.

Ryfkogel, H. A. L., 162 Post St., San Francisco. T.

Sadler, Lena K., 32 N. State St., Chicago. 8, 1.

Sanes, K. I., 519 Jenkins Bldg., Pittsburgh. 4, 6, 7, 9, 0, 2, 3, 4.

Sandow, B. F., Dalziel Bldg., Oakland, Calif. 5.

Sanes, K. I., 515 Jenkins Bldg., Pittsburgh. T.

Sarles, W. T., Sparta, Wis. T.

Saunders, Orris W., 1700 Broadway, Camden, N. J. 4.

Sawyer, Chas. J., Windsor, N. C. 9, 2.

Sawyer, M. H., 401 Central Life Bldg., Ottawa, Ill. 3.

Seashore, D. E., 403 Central Ave., Duluth, Minn. 3.

Seibert, Simmons M., Wenatchee, Wash. 5.

Shann, Herman, 207 Hart St., Brooklyn. 2.

Schaeffer, C. D., 26-28 N. 8th St., Allentown, Pa. 2.

Schenck, B. R., 1337 D. Whitney Bldg., Detroit. 8, 9, 2.

Schmeling, A. F., Columbus, Wis. 9, 0, 3.

Schmitz, Henry, 25 E. Washington St., Chicago. 4, 5.

Scholl, Albert J., 1336 S. Main St., Los Angeles. 1, 5.

Schumann, Edward A., 15 Pelham Rd., Philadelphia. 2, 6, 9, 4.

Schwarz, Henry, 440 N. Newstead Ave., St. Louis. 9, 0, 2, 3, 4.

Schwarz, Otto Henry, 440 N. Newstead Ave., St. Louis. 4.

Scull, Wm. B., 3024 Richmond St., Philadelphia. 9, 1, 2, 3.

Seippel, Clara P., 2300 Michigan Ave., Chicago. 3.

Sellers, Ira J., 607 Empire Bldg., Birmingham, Ala. T.

Seymour, F. E., Fort Dodge, Ia. 3.

Sexton, J. C., Rushville, Ind. 1.

Shafer, H. O., 1200 N. Dearborn St., Chicago. 0, 3.

Shea, William E., Hammond Blk., Missoula, Mont. 5.

Shedd, G. H., N. Conway, N. H. T.

Shedd, J. Z., N. Conway, N. H. T.

Sherrick, C., Monmouth, Ill. 3.

Sherwood, H. H., Humboldt, S. D. 3.

Sherwood, W. A., 289 Garfield Place, Brooklyn. T.

Shimer, Sterling D., 120 N. 3d St., Easton, Pa. 9, 2, 4.

Shoemaker, G. E., 3727 Chestnut St., Philadelphia. 4, 6, 7, 9, 0, 2, 4.

Shrom, Ralph E., 1745 N. 17th St., Philadelphia. 4.

Shulean, N. S., Cambridge, Minn. 3.

Silver, H. M., 276 Madison Ave., New York. T.

Simpson, Abbie Winegar, 10th and Linden St., Long Beach, Calif. 1.

Simpson, F. F., 7th floor Jenkins rcade Bldg., ttsbur . 4, 6, A 9, 0, 1, 2, 3 P.. gh

Sivertsen, Ivar, 3404 10th Ave., S., Minneapolis. 3.

Skeel, Donald W., 1236 Merchants Nat. Bank Bldg., Los Angeles. 1.

Slemons, J. Morris, 3404 Clay St., San Francisco. 5.

Slocumb, Maude S., 3535 Fremont Ave., N., Minneapolis. 8, 3.

Small, W. B., 2232 Green St., Philadelphia. 9, 4.

Smith, A. J., 815 N. 5th St., Leavenworth, Kan. 3, 4.

mith, A. M., Paris, Ark. T.

mith, Chas. J., 1006 Broadway Bldg., Portland, Ore. 5.

Smith, Clarence A., 719 Cobb Bldg., Seattle. 5.

Smith, Dudley, Hotel Oakland, Oakland, Calif. T.

Smith, D. Edmund, 404-6 Reid Corner, Minneapolis. T.

Smith, Hardy T., 161 W. Ind. St., Pomona, Calif. 5.

Smith, Jos. J., 325 13th Ave., Newark, N. J. 4.

Smith, J. J., Paris, Ark. T.

Smith, J. L., Williston, S. C. 4.

Smith, L. W., 6024 Station St., E. Pittsburgh. 4.

Smith, Mary A., 33 Newberry St., Boston. 3, 5.

mith, Norman M., 3010 Hennepin Ave., Minneapolis. 3.

Smith, P. Albert, 213 Main St., Faribault, Minn. 3.

Smith, Richard R., Metz Bldg., Grand Rapids, Mich. 9, 0, 1, 2, 3.

Smith, W. J., Cadillac, Mich. 5

Snow Frank W., 24 Essex, Newburyport, Mass. T.

Sohmer, A. E., Mankato, Minn. T.

Somers, George B., 2662 Vallejo St., San Francisco. 5, 1, 2, 3.

Souder, Carl L., Columbia City, Ind. 5.

Southmayd, Le Roy, 207 Ford Bldg., Great Falls, Mont. 4, 5.

Southworth, H. E., Wright & Callender Bldg., Los Angeles. 5.

Spaeth, Wm. L. C., 5000 Jackson St., Philadelphia. 4.

Spalding, Alfred Baker, Lane Hosp., San Francisco. 3, 5.

Speik, Frederick A., 800 Auditorium, Los Angeles. T.

Spelman, James F., Anaconda, Mont. T.

Sperry, Mary A., 240 Stockton St., San Francisco. 5.

Spiller, Wm. H., 307 Second Ave., New York City. 9, 1, 2.

Spiro, Harry, 742 Hyde St., San Francisco. 5.

Sprecher, S., Tripp, S. D. 3, 4.

Sprigg, W. M., The Rochambeau, Washington, D. C. 4, 8, 2.

Springer, Willard, 810 Washington St., Wilmington, Del. 2.

Spurlock, G. H., 3217 Austin St., Houston, Tex. 3.

Spurney, A. B., Reserve Trust Bank Bldg., Cleveland. 2, 3, 4.

Spurney, A. F., 403 Osborn Bldg., Cleveland. 9, 2, 3, 4.

Stahl, Alfred, 565 Bergen St., Newark, N. J. 9, 2.

Stamm, Camille J., 1412 Diamond St., Philadelphia. 4.

Staples, A. H., 1739 S. St., N.W., Washington, D. C. 2, 4.

Stark, Bertha 516 Sutter St., San Fra

tark, Sigmar, 1108 McMillan St., Cincinnati. 4.

Stealy, J. H., Freeport, Ill. T.

Stein, Arthur, 11 E. 68th St., New York City. 9, 2.

Stelle, H. L., 502½ Broadway, Pittsburg, Kan. 1.

Stevens, R. George, Boyce-Greeley Bldg., Sioux Falls, S. D. T.

Stevenson, Herbert E., 620 N. Oregon St., El Paso, Texas. 5.

Stewart, W. S., 98 S. Franklin St., Wilkes-Barre, Pa. T.

Stillians, Daniel C., 414 W. Colton Ave., Redlands, Calif. 1.

Stillwagen, Chas. A., 1212 Highland Bldg., Pittsburgh. 2.

Stimson, Cheney M., 1801 Cayuga St., Philadelphia. 4.

Stoeltzing, C. A., 759 E. 105th St., Cleveland. 2, 3.

Stone, I. S., Stoneleigh Ct., Washington, D. C. 4, 6, 7, 8, 9, 4.

Stowell, J. H., 2633 Indiana Ave., Chicago. T.

Strasser, August A., Arlington, N. J. 7, 9, 4, 5.

Strauss, S., 440 West End Ave., New York. T.

Strobell, C. W., 17 E. 38th St., New York. T.

Stubbs, H. J., 1204 Delaware Ave., Wilmington, Del. 2, 4.

Stuckert, Harry, 2116 N. 21st St., Philadelphia. 4.

Sturmdorf, Arnold, 51 W. 74th St., New York City. 2.

Sullivan, W. G., 319 Prairie Ave., Providence, R. I. 6, 8, 0, 4.

Sundin, P. O., 1516 Girard St., Los Angeles. 3, 5.

Sutherland, J., 605 Old Nat. Bk. Bldg., Spokane, Wash. T.

Sutton, Frederic A., 112 Day St., Orange, N. J. 4.

Sutton, F. M., 1101 Empire Life Bldg., Atlanta, Ga. 4.

Sutton, H. T., 37 S. 6th St., Zanesville, Ohio. 0, 3.

Swahlen, P. H., St. Ann's Asylum, St. Louis. 8, 9, 0, 1.

Swift, John B., Jr., 419 Beacon St., Boston. 2.

Talley, D. F., 1808 7th Ave., Birmingham, Ala. T.

Taneyhill, G. Lane, 1103 Madison Ave., Baltimore. 9, 2, 4.

Taussig, Fred J., 4506 Maryland Ave., St. Louis. 5, 6, 8, 0, 2, 3.

Taylor, H. C., 32 W. 50th St., New York City. 2, 5.

Taylor, Wm. W., Randolph Bldg., Memphis, Tenn. 4.

Teass, Chester J., 210 Post St., San Francisco. 5.

Tebbetts, Hiram B., 618 Trust & Savings Bldg., Los Angeles. 1.

Teel, A. W., 343 S. Brand St., Glendale, Calif. 1.

Telford, A. T., 124 S. Fair St., Olney, Ill. 2.

Teller, Wm. H., 1713 Green St., Philadelphia. T.

Thienhaus, C. O., 883 Cambridge Ave., Milwaukee. 8, 2, 3.

Thomas, Geo. E., 1. E. Lake St., Minneapolis. 3.

Thomas, G. N., 3601 Montana St., El Paso, Texas. 5.

Thomas, H. H., Decorah, Iowa. 3.

Thomas, J. J., 1110 Euclid Ave., Cleveland. 5.

Thompson, A. S., Mt. Horeb, Wis. 3.

Thomson, Charles E., Scranton Private Hosp., Scranton, Pa. T.

Thompson, Chas. O., 589 Beacon St., Boston. T.

Thompson, Harry F., Forest City, Iowa. 3.

Thompson, Wm. M., 512 Wrightwood Ave., Chicago. 4.

Thornby, H. J., Barnesville, Minn. 3.

Thorpe, John N., 1637 W. 51st St., Chicago. 3, 4.

Throckmorton, Jeanette F., Chariton, Iowa. 3, 4.

Tobias, John B., 305 E. Northampton Ave., Wilkes-Barre, Pa. 5.

Todd, Frank L., 804 Sherman Ave., Pittsburgh. 4.

Tompkins, Christopher, 116 E. Franklin St., Richmond, Va. 5, 6, 1.

Tophan, Edw., 126 Stockton St., San Francisco. 5.

Torbert, James R., 252 Marlborough St., Boston. T.

Townsend, Mary E., 13 S. Pennsylvania Ave., Atlantic City, N. J. 9, 2, 4.

Towslee, L. G., 8118 Carnegie Ave., Cleveland. 2.

Tracy, S. E., 1527 Spruce St., Philadelphia. 4, 9, 2, 4.

Trask, Chas. D., 1713 Lathrop Bldg., Kansas City, Mo. 2, 3.

Treichler, Elsie R., 1721 N. 33d St., Philadelphia. 4.

Trigg, J. M., 516 Metropolitan Bldg., St. Louis. T.

Trueheart, M., Sterling, Kan. 4.

Trueman, J. E., Garden City Bank Bldg., San Jose, Calif. 1.

Truesdale, Philemon E., 1820 Highland Ave., Fall River, Mass. 3.

Truex, Edw. H., 802 Main St., East Hartford, Conn. 4.

Twitchell, Herbert F., 10 Pine St., Portland, Me. T.

Twombly, E. L., 416 Marlborough St., Boston. T.

Ulrich, Mabel S., 420 Syndicate Bldg., Minneapolis. 3.

Van Dyke, J. H., Cedar Falls, Iowa. 3.

Van Fleet, Edw. A., 210 McCaque Bldg., Omaha, Neb. 2, 5.

Van Gaasbeek, C. H., 29 Berkeley St., Springfield, Mass. T.

Van Hoosen, Bertha, 4845 Calumet Ave., Chicago. 3, 4.

Van Orden, Kate P., 1125 Paru St., Alameda, Calif. 5.

Van Tine, Cochran, Boulder Creek, Calif. 5.

St., San Pedro,

Vineberg, Hiram N., 751 Madison Ave., New York City. 2.

Von der Lieth, H. O., 634 Powell St., San Francisco. 1, 5.

Voorhess, Harry M., 1005 Brockman Bldg., Los Angeles. 5.

Vowinckel, F. W., 1200 Octavia St., San Francisco. 1, 5.

Wade, H. A., 495 Greene Ave., Brooklyn. 2.

Wadsworth, Richard G., 522 Commonwealth Ave., Boston. 3.

Wahrer, Carl W., Box 211, Ft. Madison, Iowa. 3, 4.

Waiss, A. S., Keystone Apt., Wash. & Hyde Sts., San Francisco. 5.

Wakefield, W. F. B., 1525 Sutter St., San Francisco. 2, 5.

Walker, E., 712 S. 4th St., Evansville, Ind. 4, 9, 0, 1, 2, 3, 4.

Walker, Frank B., 402 Washington Arcade, Detroit. T.

Walker, J. A., Whitaker Bldg., Rms. 1, 2, Shawnee, Okla. T.

Walker, J. E., Hornell, N. Y. T.

Wallace, W. L., 720 S. Crouse Ave., Syracuse, N. Y. T.

Wanous, Ernest Z., 2425 S. Irving Ave., Minneapolis. 3.

Ward, G. G., Jr., 71 W. 50th St., New York City. 4, 6, 7, 9, 4.

Warham, T. T., 402 Masonic Temple, Minneapolis. 3.

Waring, T. P., 10 Taylor St., W., Savannah, Ga. T.

Waterworth, S. J., 102 S. 2d St., Clearfield, Pa. T.

Watkins, T. J., 5436 East End Ave., Chicago. 2.

Watson, W. C., 446 Stratford Ave., Bridgeport, Conn. 4.

Waugh, Justin M., Hood River, Ore. T.

Webb, M. S., 224 S. 5th St., Cedar Rapids, Iowa. 3.

Weber, A. L., Cucumonga, Calif. 1.

Weber, Geo. T., Olney, Ill. 9, 2.

Weir, C. F., 63d and Stewart Ave., Chicago. 2, 4, 5.

Weir, Wm. H., 1021 Prospect Ave., Cleveland. 4.

Weiss, Edward A., 1804 Wightman St., Pittsburgh. 6, 8, 9, 4.

Welpton, H. G., Citizens Bank Bldg., Des Moines, Iowa. 4.

Welsh, Prudence M., 345 E. Ocean Ave., Long Beach, Calif. 1.

Werner, O. S.,
Weston, C. G., 2107
S., Minneapolis. 3.
Westerfeld, Otto F., 240 Stockton
St., San Francisco. 5.
Westmoreland, W. P., 443 Trust
Co. of Ga. Bldg., Atlanta, Ga. T.
Wetherill, H. G., 1127 Race St.,
Denver. 4, 7, 8, 0, 1, 2, 5.
Wheat, A. F., Dunlap Block, Man-
chester, N. H. 1.
Whery, Mary A., Ft. Wayne, Ind.
4.
White, Allan S., Rice Lake, Wis. 3.
White, Frank, 1302 W. Broad St.,
Philadelphia. T.
White, Sherman T., Redding, Calif.
5.
White, Wm. K., 1819 N. Charles
St., Baltimore. 4.
Whitehead, H. E., 5 Washington
St., Mt. Holly, N. J. 2.
Wiatt, W. S., 4 Lewis Place, St.
Louis. T.
Wickstrom, Albert M., 1254 Addi-
son St., Chicago. 5.
Widdowson, F. R., 1438 N. 60th
St., Philadelphia. 2, 4.
Wiggins, L. J. L., 11½ N. Main St.,
E. St. Louis, Ill. T.
Wilkes, Benjamin A., Met. Bldg.,
St. Louis. 5.
Williams, Alice B., Columbia City,
Ind. 4.
Williams, Henry L., 616 Donaldson
Bldg., Minneapolis. 3.
Williams, Philip F., 121 S. 20th St.,
Philadelphia. 4.
Williamson, W. L., 628 Goodwyn
Bldg., Memphis, Tenn. 4.
Willits, Emma K., 391 Sutter St.,
San Francisco. 1, 3, 5.

Willmoth, A. D., Masonic Bldg.,
Louisville, Ky. 2, 4, 5.
Wilson, Carl G. W., 1st Natl. Bank
Bldg., Palo Alto, Calif. 1.
Wilson, Dora Green, 626 Lathrop
Bldg., Kansas City, Mo. 0, 1.
Wilson, J. Miller, 1242 E. Colorado
St., Pasadena, Calif. 1.
Wilson, R. A., Odessa, Texas. T.
Wilson, Warren, Northfield, Minn.
3.
Wilson, W. F., 120 Lyon Ave., Lake
City, Minn. 3.
Wiltsie, S. F., 811 Cobb Bldg.,
Seattle. T.
Windmueller, E., Woodstock, Ill. 3.
Winebrake, A. J., 608 N. Main
Ave., Scranton, Pa. 9, 2, 4.
Wiseman, B. W. S., Culver, Ind. 4.
Witherbee, O. O., 1020 Burlington
Ave., Los Angeles. 5.
Wobus, R. E., 2406 Kingshighway,
St. Louis. 8, 9, 0, 2, 3.
Wood, Everett A., Maywood Hosp.,
Sedalia, Mo. 4.
Wright, George I., 5th & Main Sts.,
Klamath, Ore. 5.
Yarros, R. S., 800 S. Halsted St.,
Chicago. 3.
Yates, H. Wellington, 1229 D. Whit-
ney Bldg., Detroit. 4.
Young, E. Weldon, Cobb Bldg.,
Seattle. 5.
Young, J. R., Berkley Bldg., Ander-
son, S. C. 4.
Young, S. J., Valparaiso, Ind. T.
Youngs, Alfred H., 7 Hyde Bldg.,
Pierre, S. D. 3.
Zimmerman, G. A., 1407 Market
St., Harrisburg, Pa. 4.
Zinke, E. Gustav, 4 W. 7th St.,
Cincinnati. 0, 2, 3, 4.

INDEX

Lightning Source UK Ltd.
Milton Keynes UK
UKHW010613120219
337137UK00007B/1388/P